"Carol Olmert has made a major contribution paruresis (shy bladder syndrome). Her comprehensive book provides practical, clear, effective information on understanding and recovering from the condition. While explicitly written for women, anyone can benefit from reading her work; sufferers, clinicians, and support people will find this an invaluable resource."

Carl Robbins, MS, MEd, NCC, LCPC
Director of Training, Anxiety & Stress Disorders Institute of Maryland
International Paruresis Association Co-Founder

"I didn't realize this could be such a problem," a physician once told me. That quote came to my mind after reading this excellent book. I especially like the biographical accounts; also the technical detail of catheter usage for severely unreliable urinary systems is a green flag to me of this book's accuracy. Bravo Carol – what a blessing this book is for women and men struggling to overcome paruresis!"

Phil Baumgaertner
Former International Paruresis Association President

"Finally, a book that talks about the taboo subject of paruresis. Carol Olmert's book is a well written, thoughtful and serious exploration of paruresis, which is a disorder that has caused endless suffering and shame among the millions of women with this affliction. Therapists will find the information provided informative and instructive and those that suffer from this debilitating disorder will not only find solace in knowing they are not alone but step-by-step instructions on how to overcome this disorder. A must for all therapists' bookshelves!"

Ruth Lippin, LMSW
New York, New York

"In *Bathrooms Make Me Nervous*, Carol Olmert delivers a thorough, clear and accessible guide for women who struggle with urination anxiety, otherwise known as paruresis. Olmert's work offers more than a "how to" for women with this problem. In reading this guide anyone involved in the life of a woman with this issue will gain an authentic understanding of their loved one's struggle. Most importantly, Carol Olmert presents a message of hope. A MUST READ for all concerned about paruresis."

Philip Haber, MS
Former International Paruresis Association Vice President

Bathrooms Make Me Nervous

A Guidebook for Women with Urination Anxiety (Shy Bladder)

Carol Olmert

CJOB Publications
Walnut Creek, CA

Publisher's Note

The information provided in this book is general in nature and is intended for educational and informational purposes only. It is not meant to replace or substitute for the evaluation, judgment, diagnosis, and medical or preventive treatment of a physician or other health care professional. The author makes no representations concerning the efficacy, appropriateness or suitability of any products, medications, or treatments discussed, nor is she responsible for the contents of any linked site or any link contained in a linked site, or any changes or updates to such sites.

Links to websites contained in this book can be found at
http://www.bathroomsmakemenervous.com

Cover design by Bonnie Matza

Printed in the United States of America

Library of Congress Control Number: 2008904562
ISBN 978-0-6152-4024-4

This book is dedicated to those women
with Shy Bladder Syndrome
who have allowed me into their lives
by sharing their stories.

Acknowledgements

Dr. Steve Soifer's and his co-authors' pioneering work on *Shy Bladder Syndrome: Your Step-by-Step Guide to Overcoming Paruresis* made this book possible.

Special acknowledgements to Drs. Steve Flannes and Frank Barham, Jeri Holman, Reva Brodsky, and to the late Alice Barham and Joyce Kaplan, whose belief in me and this project has been resolute; to Dr. Richard Ziprin, Carl Robbins, and Phil Baumgaertner who have helped to take me and countless others out of the (water) closet; to Drs. Jerry Donchin, Mel Friedman, Alex Gardner, Dharmini Harichandran, Howard Liebgold, and Alan Tobias, whose feedback and affirmation enabled me to complete this book.

I gratefully wish to recognize Lynn and Sylvia, my original "pee buddies," who paved the way for me; Roz Parenti and Ruth Lippin for their invaluable assistance and words of wisdom; the International Paruresis Association Board of Directors (current and former), moderators of and contributors to the IPA Discussion Board; and all members and friends of the IPA who continue to provide me with encouragement and inspiration.

My sincere thanks to Andrea Weyant, Sharon Sipprell, Susan Stanwick, and especially Barbara Templeton for their editorial guidance and much gratitude to Ericka Hamburg, Susan Hillyard, and Bonnie Matza for their artistic contributions.

My deepest love and appreciation go to my husband, Alan Burckin, MD, my family, and my many friends who relentlessly offer both practical and emotional support.

Table of Contents

Foreword

In her book, *Bathrooms Make Me Nervous: A Guidebook for Women with Urination Anxiety (Shy Bladder)*, Carol Olmert has written a crucial and much needed guide for women suffering from paruresis, or shy bladder syndrome. Until now, there have only been a few publications on the subject: a general book, a book for men, and a book of recovery stories. Her book adds to the literature in an important, accessible, and well-written way.

From her own personal experience in recovery (which includes helping to co-lead several IPA-sponsored all-women's workshops) to her extensive knowledge of the subject matter, Ms. Olmert has put together a well-grounded personal manual to help empower women along their own paths of self-recovery.

Perhaps most importantly, Ms. Olmert goes to great lengths to cover the latest treatment methods available for paruresis, some of which have not been discussed in print before. This section will be helpful for women and men alike. In particular, the "breath-holding" technique is highlighted, which holds new hope for people with paruresis. Moreover, she provides many practical suggestions, including resources for traveling, alternatives to bathroom use, and a good discussion of many of the current issues that affect the paruretic community.

On a personal note, Ms. Olmert has been a long-time friend and supporter of the IPA. She has served on the organization's board for many years and helped its growth in numerous ways.

Steven Soifer, PhD, LGSW
Co-founder and CEO, International Paruresis Association
Author, *The Shy Bladder Syndrome:
Your Step-By-Step Guide to Overcoming Paruresis*

Preface

This book is written for women who find it hard to urinate in bathrooms when others are nearby or who avoid using public restrooms altogether.

Most people take the process of urination for granted as a natural, normal part of their daily existence. A minority of women and men – an estimated 7% of the U.S. population – are bathroom-challenged. They have fears that interfere with their ability to use public or private restrooms.

Some women put up with their problem, diminishing its importance in their lives or developing daily routines to accommodate it. Others, including those who cannot produce a urine specimen on demand as a prerequisite to being hired or staying employed, face the consequence of loss of work.

Many are simply unaware that they have a treatable condition, a type of social anxiety disorder called *paruresis*, or in the vernacular better known as *shy bladder* or *bashful bladder*.

Those who do seek professional help from physicians and mental health specialists often encounter ignorance, skepticism, or denial. Many health care practitioners simply lack knowledge about the very existence or validity of this condition. They are just not equipped to address its physical and psychological components.

In their groundbreaking book, *Shy Bladder Syndrome: Your Step-by-Step Guide to Overcoming Paruresis*, Dr. Steven Soifer and his colleagues explore this affliction in depth. Since its publication in 2001, thousands of people have realized they are not flawed for life, and many have recovered to the extent that paruresis no longer dominates it.

A book for women

Bathrooms Make Me Nervous: A Guidebook for Women with Urination Anxiety (Shy Bladder) is unique because it focuses on women who suffer from paruresis.

o If you're new to this subject, find out if you meet the criteria for having this condition.

- o If you're already familiar with paruresis, you will find various strategies that other women (me included) have employed in order to cope.
- o Learn the implications of the differences between women's and men's bathroom behavior.
- o Discover how to challenge and change your thinking patterns about bathrooms and the people you may encounter in them.
- o Explore treatment methods that will allow you to recover.
- o Read real life stories and anecdotes from other women who have managed and recovered from paruresis.

A personal journey

For more than 40 years, I suffered from a severe case of paruresis. Almost every waking moment my attention was focused on everyday rituals – the when, where, how and whether I could urinate that day and the consequences of not being able to do so. When am I going to find that next safe bathroom? If I'm thirsty, can I risk drinking something now?

As a result, I missed out on all kinds of life-affirming activities and opportunities. In short, my condition ran my life – it defined who I was to a large degree – and I felt very alone and isolated because of it.

My journey from being a severe paruretic to living a paruresis-free life led me to write this book. The path was not linear. It required a test of faith, change in mindset, and determination to succeed at any cost.

Big changes

Since my recovery, my life has changed in many positive ways. I have taken a lot of risks, grown in confidence, and increased my resolve to help other women recover from paruresis. I have served on the Board of Directors of the International Paruresis Association (IPA), respond to queries from female paruretics across the globe, and co-facilitated two All-Female Paruretics' IPA Workshops.

In *Bathrooms Make Me Nervous*, I provide you with the wisdom that I and other women have gained from our personal experiences with this condition.

You will learn that there is nothing wrong with you. You will learn you are not alone. You will come to learn to appreciate yourself. You will learn to change habits that have been detrimental to your well-being.

By writing this book for female paruretics and those who wish to support them, it is my deepest desire that you will find inspiration and encouragement to undertake or continue your quest for recovery.

Introduction

I had become a prisoner of My Own Private Bathroom, a sanctuary and source of salvation in my life, and I was desperate to be released from a life-long sentence.

For over 40 years, since I was 13 and at a familiar summer camp, I could not urinate easily while other people were nearby in a bathroom. It didn't matter whether it was a women's public restroom, the home of my friends and relatives or even in my own home if visitors were close by or someone was waiting for me. I simply could not "go" at will when I needed to, no matter how hard I tried.

Despite my limitations in being unable to urinate "like everyone else," I resisted my temptation to surrender to paruresis. Instead, I continued to try and live my life as best as I could. I simply rationalized away my condition and accepted my fate and circumstances. *"Some people,"* I told myself, *"are in wheelchairs, while others are blind. They manage; you can, too."*

In the most desperate of times, I prayed.

The mind-body connection

After my initial episode, my fears about urinating and the consequences of not being able to intensified. The urologists to whom my well-meaning parents took me performed a variety of medical tests, some of which were quite painful. No physiological cause was ever found. One urologist reassured my mother by telling her, *"The problem will go away once she gets married."* Another placed me on anti-anxiety medication to help relieve stress.

The pattern of avoidance of bathrooms had set in, and my condition essentially took on a life of its own. When I was heavily stressed and/or afraid, the tension I felt was channeled to and registered in my pelvic region. It became the repository for the expression of powerful emotions: anger, fear, even excitement. The sphincter muscles, which govern the release of urine, shut down, rendering it impossible for me to urinate except through catheterization or in the privacy of my home without anyone present.

Bathroom blues

The interior of my mind contained a constellation of restrictive thoughts that fed upon each other. Entering a bathroom, I would constantly think: "Who will see me? Who will hear me? Who is waiting to use it? And what might they be saying about me?" My heart pounded whenever I even dared to approach. The anticipation of failure before I entered a restroom set the tone for my experience. When I could not perform, I would beat myself up emotionally.

On a day-to-day basis, I coped for years by holding in my urine for long periods, refrained from drinking liquids, made sure I urinated at home before leaving, and excelled at locating unoccupied or single-occupancy public bathrooms.

When I was unable to urinate after a very long period of time, I resorted to catheterization – a process in which a sterile tube is temporarily inserted into the opening of the urethra to allow urine to flow out automatically. Medical personnel or friends performed this process for me until I learned to do it myself many years later. Catheterization was the only sure-fire method of which I was aware for finding immediate relief.

As the years wore on, my coping strategies began to expire. My bladder capacity, for example, diminished over time, and I could no longer hold my urine for excessive hours without feeling pain. Even after a successful catheterization, I often could not relax my bladder muscles enough to urinate on my own, sometimes for periods of up to three days.

My constricted life: Why me?

My fears and steady stream of obsessive thoughts resulted in my daily life becoming severely restricted. I constructed it around the presence or absence of bathroom facilities – and the people I might encounter in them. I missed out on all kinds of activities and opportunities: sleepovers, proms, sharing a ski cabin, backpacking in the wilds, any lengthy social or business engagement, travel, and many, many more. When asked to produce a urine specimen for a medical examination, I failed every time. In short, I felt paralyzed.

Even though I told my family and some friends about my distress, I felt alone and misunderstood, embarrassed and hopeless. The serious emotional toll that was exacted was just as debilitating as the physical discomfort. My self-esteem and self-confidence were eroded.

Gradually, over a period of time as my condition progressively worsened, I learned to avoid using public restrooms almost altogether and finally reached a point where I was afraid to leave my home with My Own Private Bathroom for more than a few hours at a time.

Why me? Why can't I be *"normal?"* What "caused" my problem, and how could I overcome it? As a researcher by profession, I felt compelled to find answers to my nagging questions. Over the course of many years, I consulted with a host of urologists, psychologists, psychiatrists, and social workers. I experimented with different kinds of techniques, such as biofeedback, meditation, hypnotherapy, gestalt, bioenergetics, acupuncture, visualizations, and the like.

No person or technique helped because the nature of my condition was misunderstood. Though well-intended, these health care professionals lacked the awareness that social anxiety disorders like mine respond well to one particular kind of short-term therapy called Cognitive-Behavioral.

A moment of tearful hope

In 1997, I made a startling discovery that ultimately changed the course of my life. I located an Internet-based Discussion Forum (now operated by the International Paruresis Association or IPA (www.paruresis.org). Here I found others with my symptoms, mostly men, who communicated and commiserated. I felt as if I had just found a lifeboat full of survivors from the same nightmare.

Tearful but overjoyed, I readily absorbed some basic information about my disorder and its effect on others. I learned that my condition:

o Actually has a medical name – paruresis (par-you-ree-sis) – but is often more commonly referred to as "shy bladder" or "bashful bladder" syndrome. (Other names include "pee shyness" and the more technical term, "psychogenic urinary retention").

o Is considered a *performance*-based anxiety, or type of social anxiety condition, much like public speaking or the fear of eating or drinking in public. The person is usually, but not always, shy and fears being scrutinized or criticized by others when performing in public – in this case, urinating while in a restroom. The *Diagnostic and Statistical Manual of Mental Disorders IV* (DSM) categorizes paruresis as a social anxiety disorder, diagnostic code 300.23 (American Psychiatric Association, 1994).

o Is one shared by many others – perhaps as many as 7% of the U.S. population (Soifer, 2001; Malouff, 1985). According to a sub-analysis of the 1997 National Co-Morbidity Study, 6.7% of a random sample of people in the United States said that they have difficulty urinating when away from home (Kessler, et al., 1998). Many of those are people with paruresis. Of those, a significant number are, like I was, critically impaired to the extent that their symptoms heavily interfere with their relationships, work, and travel.

o Affects both men and women alike – but is more often recognized among men. Many of us are highly sensitive people who are intelligent, good, kind, and empathetic – people with qualities to be celebrated. We are simply bathroom-challenged individuals who have difficulty urinating under certain circumstances.

o Is often kept a big secret by people who have it, usually out of shame and embarrassment.

o Often goes unrecognized by well-meaning physicians and other health care practitioners who may be ignorant about its existence, resulting in faulty diagnoses and poor referrals.

o Is the central focus of The International Paruresis Association (IPA) (www.paruresis.org), a nonprofit organization whose mission it is to help paruretics (those with paruresis) overcome the stigma, embarrassment, and isolation associated with the condition. The IPA also sponsors workshops to help sufferers overcome their condition and facilitates the establishment of support or self-help groups around the world.

And the best news is that this disorder...

is treatable with a variety of approaches, including psychotherapy, medication, and support group work, or a combination thereof. No one treatment is effective for everyone.

One highly effective approach has been through exposure-based Cognitive-Behavioral Therapy (CBT), a process that allows a slow and gradual recovery – like climbing the rungs of a ladder one step at a time.

o The **cognitive** part helps identify and then alter distorted thoughts and attitudes regarding bathrooms and the people in them. For example, "People will think I am weird if I am sitting in a stall and they do not hear me urinate."

o The **behavioral** component utilizes the practice of desensitization techniques through which you learn to gradually expose yourself to (rather than *avoid*) increasingly difficult situations in which you find it difficult to urinate.

Chapter 9 covers CBT in greater depth.

My journey toward recovery

Simply put, I wanted my life back, and I was willing to tolerate all of the anxiety it took to reclaim it.

Supported by members and leaders of the IPA, both men and women, I began a journey toward a goal of complete recovery from paruresis, a passage that is a privilege to share with you.

It was clear to me that there was no "quick fix," no "cure," nor any pill or herbal supplement I could swallow to magically eliminate my symptoms. Rather, I knew I had to totally commit to a treatment program that would help me overcome paruresis.

I wasn't quite psychologically ready to enroll in recovery workshops that were being offered by the IPA. Other events intervened that caused me great anxiety, sleepless nights, and panic attacks – a lumpectomy, pressure at work, and a crisis in my personal life. Very depressed, depleted, and at a low point, I consulted with a psychiatrist who prescribed Prozac™, an antidepressant, to stabilize my mood. Though highly resistant to taking it because of the stigma attached, I did because I had little choice. The psychiatrist also offered me something equally important – *hope*.

Six weeks later, the black clouds started to dissipate as the medication took effect. Many of my obsessive thoughts about urinating or not urinating faded. In a more relaxed state, I was able to cultivate a ho-hum attitude: "It's fine if I urinate; fine if I don't. I will not be concerned about the outcome."

I went on to enroll in two IPA workshops, at which I made tremendous progress, step by step. Some of the basic and valuable lessons I learned:

o When it comes to urinating, there are no such things as "successes" or "failures" (the IPA calls them "misfires"). The success is in the practice, not the outcome.

o In order to recover, I had to let myself experience firsthand the terrible anxiety that results from not urinating, feeling all those uncomfortable, distressing feelings and reactions. I had to reject avoidance and face my fears. Though counter-intuitive, I had to take the risk of deliberately *not* voiding while in a bathroom so I could learn to tolerate, and ultimately conquer, the anxiety.

o I have the right – the entitlement – to stay in a stall for as long as I want or need. I count just as much as anyone else!

o I will not concern myself with what anyone else might be thinking about me when I use a restroom. Besides, they are likely to be self-absorbed, and furthermore it doesn't matter to them if I can or cannot urinate.

o The path toward recovery is not straight and consists of taking "baby steps." Some days I will make progress, other days not. I'm not having a relapse – just a more difficult day – and each time is just a new experience.

o It is not a catastrophe if I cannot urinate, even though I may be experiencing frustration, discomfort, or even pain. Even in the worst case scenario, I have alternatives, such as self-catheterization or finding relief by seeking medical attention.

Practice makes perfect

Armed with new-found confidence and dedication, I continued to practice – over and over – many of the exercises I learned at the IPA workshop. I treated recovery work like a job, which is what you must do if you are truly going to recover. I practiced a lot, with and without friends and acquaintances, exposing myself to situations I never thought possible.

What was new this time was that a switch had been activated in my brain. I actually *looked forward* to my practice sessions. I kept repeating a self-taught mantra, *"I'm a free peer (that's pee-er), and I will stake my ground here for as long as I need."* I felt a sense of power in relation to the bathroom that I had lost long ago.

No, these practice sessions weren't always fun, and, yes, sometimes they were stressful. But instead of avoiding bathrooms, I confronted them head on. I made a game out of it, one which I felt assured I could win. *"Just come and get me, world; here I am!"* became my attitude.

Little by little, I started to feel – for lack of a better word – *normal!* I wasn't consciously thinking of urinating. I assumed I would go and built on each success.

Through extensive communication with other female paruretics over the years, I also gained new insights about issues and behaviors that are unique to women. It is their highly personal revelations that, while anecdotal, have resulted in a cumulative knowledge base that forms the foundation of this book, and they're the people to whom I am especially indebted.

Coming out of the (water) closet in other areas of my life

As a result of my recovery, my life has changed in many remarkable and unforeseen ways. By completely coming out of the (water) closet, I have flourished in other areas of my life as well. (Note: For readers who may not be familiar with the term, "water closet" is a British term for toilet – as is "WC" and "loo.")

By feeling entitled to stay in a bathroom stall for as long as I like, I felt empowered – that I counted, that I was just as important as the next person. I took new risks: I got married for the first time! I became a step-grandmother! I became a much stronger person, able to face new challenges that I had formerly avoided.

Am I fully *"cured"*? No, but I have recovered to the extent that paruresis no longer controls my life. Sure, I experience hesitancy and an occasional "misfire" in certain situations, such as urinating outdoors, but probably no more so than anyone else. I no longer obsess about bathrooms, but I still carry my catheter kit with me just in case I need to get out of a difficult spot – only now it's buried at the bottom of my purse.

When I look back on my life's accomplishments, overcoming paruresis is definitely at the top of my list.

You, too, can leave the prison of Your Own Private Bathroom. You can be liberated! Let me show you how.

I wish you the best of luck.

P.S. For a more in-depth version of my personal journey toward recovery, turn to Appendix 3.

Chapter One
Do You Suffer from Paruresis?

A Self-Screening Test

Are you a woman who has difficulty using restrooms? Ask yourself some questions up front:

☐ Do you usually fear, feel very anxious about, or avoid using public restrooms while others are present?

☐ Do you continually worry that someone might see, hear, or wait for you to urinate in a bathroom?

☐ Are you concerned what other people are thinking when you are trying to urinate?

☐ Do you usually wait for others to leave the restroom before you attempt to urinate?

☐ Are you able to urinate at home when you find it difficult to or simply cannot when away?

☐ Does your avoidance of or distress about using restrooms interfere significantly with your job, social activities, travel, and/or relationships?

☐ Does your fear of using restrooms seem excessive or unreasonable to you?

☐ Has a doctor or health care professional excluded a physical cause for your difficulty in urinating in bathrooms?

Adapted from *Shy Bladder Syndrome: Your Step-by-Step Guide to Overcoming Paruresis* (Soifer, Zgourides, Himle, Pickering, 2001, p. 8).

If you answered "yes" to some or most of these questions, then you might suffer from paruresis. If only one or two questions strike home but they are extremely accurate, you might be justified in calling yourself paruretic. If you have trouble urinating in the presence – or the perceived presence – of others and do not have a problem urinating while alone or in a perceived 'private' situation, then you most likely have paruresis.

The Continuum, from Mild to Severe

Before concluding that you have paruresis, understand that you, like many people, may have trouble initiating a stream of urine from time to time. Difficult situations may include those in which you feel your personal space is being invaded, you have to produce a urine sample (especially for a drug test), and/or you try to urinate immediately following surgery. Now ask yourself:

To what extent have your symptoms disrupted your work or school in the last year?

NOT AT ALL	MILDLY			MODERATELY			SUBSTANTIALLY			EXTREMELY
0 ○	1 ○	2 ○	3 ○	4 ○	5 ○	6 ○	7 ○	8 ○	9 ○	10 ○

To what extent have your symptoms disrupted your family, social life, or travel in the last year?

NOT AT ALL	MILDLY			MODERATELY			SUBSTANTIALLY			EXTREMELY
0 ○	1 ○	2 ○	3 ○	4 ○	5 ○	6 ○	7 ○	8 ○	9 ○	10 ○

Experience and studies reveal the extent to which paruresis controls or interferes with one's life is best viewed along a spectrum ranging from mild to severe.

For some women who suffer a mild case, paruresis is little more than a nuisance or mild inconvenience, not something they see a need to overcome. They might be unaware they even have it; others might silently endure.

On the other extreme, someone with a severe case of paruresis feels intense anguish about going to the bathroom when other people are around. Fears about using restrooms turn into phobias when they interrupt one's course of enjoyment or natural flow of activities.

Bathroom Experience Varies by Individual and Situation

The environmental circumstance in which paruresis occurs varies from individual to individual.

Some women, for example, cannot urinate in a quiet two- or three-stall bathroom if anyone else is there. Others prefer large restrooms with lots of stalls and high traffic due to the anonymity factor (they don't want to be seen). Some can void in single-person bathrooms, such as in private gas stations or handicapped facilities. Others have less trouble voiding while in the presence of strangers rather than friends or family members – or vice versa. Some have difficulty performing in the presence of members of the opposite sex and others simply in strange surroundings.

Common threads

While some symptoms and also their severity vary among those afflicted, there is a consistency in anxiety and thought patterns among those with paruresis. The most frequent concerns that individuals express are about:

o Being observed.

o Being heard.

o People waiting to use the facilities, either outside the stalls or in lines outside of the restroom.

o Our companion(s) waiting for us to leave the bathroom.

o Proximity to other people, especially those we know.

o Too much or too little noise – either in a restroom facility or the noise we're making (or not making) in a stall.

o Performance in a stall.

o Telling others about our problem.

And the root of the problem – many of us with paruresis are unnecessarily concerned with what people will think about us.

Some of us also share the following characteristics:

o   Inner nervousness, tension.

o   High expectations.

o   Sensitivity to criticism.

o   Perfectionism.

o   Tendency to overreact to situations.

A large-scale international study among adult paruretic males by Russell Gibbs, a researcher from Australia, confirmed that they scored significantly higher than the general population on private self-consciousness (dwelling on negative aspects of the self as well as having an interest in self-awareness), neuroticism (tending to worry a lot), and conscientiousness (reliable and complete tasks to a high standard) (Gibbs, 2004).

Now you know you are not alone. By reading some of the personal accounts of other women who suffer from paruresis, you might gain a better perspective of where you fit along this spectrum.

Stories from Female Paruretics

Many women I have met and with whom I have corresponded have expressed deep feelings of shame and embarrassment, frustration and anger; and/or a reluctance or inability to tell other people of their condition. Some vividly expound on the paralyzing effects that paruresis has had on their lives and, consequently, their self-esteem.

A woman obsesses about her wedding day and honeymoon;
she has not told her fiancée

> I am a 23-year-old female and I have had a problem with paruresis since my early teens. I am engaged and getting married next year. This should be a happy time, but I am already stressing about the wedding day. All I can think about is how a bride usually requires one (or more) of her attendants to assist her in going to the bathroom. I know that I would never be able to go like that. And even if I left the party to try to go myself, I would feel like everyone would notice my absence and know where I was, and with all that pressure, I won't be able to go.
>
> So here I am, nine months before my wedding, feeling angry and depressed that I know I am going to have to spend the majority of that day feeling uncomfortable.

But once I get through that, I have an even bigger problem: my husband-to-be has no idea that I even have this problem. I figure I should be okay when we fall into the routine of living together. For some reason, I usually don't have a problem going when he thinks I am in the bathroom for "another reason" – showering, brushing my teeth, etc. And maybe in time I will get desensitized with him, too? (I currently live with my parents and am desensitized with them).

But my real concern is the honeymoon. When we go away for a weekend, I spend about 60% of my time with paruresis problems. How can I possibly survive a honeymoon in a strange place with us in one room with one bathroom? Am I going to have to tell him? I've never told anyone; I think it might make my condition worse if I know that he knows.

Paruresis is relatively new for her but already has taken its toll on her self-esteem

I'm 28 years old and have had paruresis for about two years. It started out of the blue. There was no painful trigger that I can remember. I find that it interferes with my life very much because I'm so preoccupied by it. I can't truly enjoy any social outings because I'm so preoccupied. I've practiced desensitization and am better than before. I can go in large washrooms, such as malls and enclosed facilities or in people's homes (if there's not someone standing right outside the door), but not in small public washrooms (if someone is there, especially if line-ups are concerned), or if there's people I know around. Basically, some situations are okay and others are not. This has affected my self-esteem very much. I feel I have no one to talk to. Only my husband knows, and he doesn't quite understand. I feel like a weirdo, although I do realize this is just a form of social anxiety.

Having curtailed many activities, she's allowed her fears to rule her life

When I was working, I had an escape bathroom. My husband is very understanding about it on trips and takes me to places with bathrooms I can use, usually with no one in them or not often visited. I still prefer an empty bathroom and though I used to occasionally go with people in the bathroom at work, now I find that it is more difficult, probably because I stopped practicing. I am safe working at home so I just don't want to deal with the paruresis anymore, though I know it is still there. I don't want to do stuff anymore that frightens me either. Why put myself through that hell, the anxiety, fear... how can I enjoy doing anything when all I think about is where will I find a bathroom I can use?

Other Unfortunate Tales Abound

Maria is a victim of obsessive thinking

My needs are for privacy, having many stalls, no one waiting for me, noise is helpful, impossible to go on an airplane, always thinking about where the bathroom is, etc. I have found that my obsessive thoughts influence everything I do and do not do. I'm so worried about where the bathroom is and whether I can go.

Elena worries about the consequences of not being able to urinate

During normal day-to-day settings I don't have a problem – no problem with familiar bathrooms at work as long as they are empty, and I usually use the bathroom before I leave the house if I'm going out for dinner or a movie. But when I do go out, I constantly worry "what if I have to go...." which of course makes you HAVE to go and you know you won't be able to, etc.

Linda has trouble urinating around immediate family members

My current perception of my situation is that it is mild/nonexistent to severe depending on the circumstances. I have little to no difficulty in large restrooms with lots of stalls and high traffic. However, I experience the greatest challenge around immediate family members (who tend to be critical) and in small restrooms where even the presence of a solitary 'stranger' is inhibiting to me.

Maggie is otherwise an outgoing person

I am 21 and I have had trouble going to the bathroom in the presence of others for as long as I can remember. Just when I think I am getting better at it, I am getting worse. It is really starting to affect my life. I am a very outgoing, fun person, but I feel I am starting to not want to go out as much because I can't pee, and when I do, I am on a mission to find the perfect private bathroom.

Another Recurring Theme: Hampered Work Lives

Susan has had to live near her workplace

My paruresis worsened significantly during college and throughout my 20s – it has, of course, had a tremendous negative impact upon my entire life, including my career path (I have several times lived very near my workplace so as to be able to get home at lunch, etc.), social interactions, and my ability to travel comfortably, e.g., I sometimes experience tremendous discomfort on long airline flights and usually take my own car on trips and drive alone. And I have, of course, also engaged in many, many bathroom avoidance behaviors over the years.

After she quit her job, Michelle couldn't even urinate at home

At age 34, I have had the problem as long as I can remember and have had a lot of bladder infections in my life, probably from excessive holding. I'm immune to some antibiotics now. Sometimes it's just an inconvenience, like at my work where I can go if no one is in there. Otherwise I just wait until it's empty (two stalls). But I have quit a job, a place where I worked and peed under the same conditions for two years until I had some personal problems and suddenly couldn't go there any more, no way. That's when I couldn't even go at home. I would worry the phone was going to ring or someone would knock on the door.

Experts in the study of paruresis acknowledge that the similarities between female and male sufferers far outweigh the differences between the genders in terms of "cause," trigger events, privacy issues, and underlying psychological profiles.

Yet, some distinctions exist between men and women with respect to bathroom facility design, behavior patterns and attitudes, clothing, and also the process of self-catheterization itself. As a result of these differences, coping mechanisms vary between the sexes, and treatment methods need to be adapted accordingly.

Why Does Paruresis Seem to Affect Men More?

Theoretically speaking, women are equally as disposed to having paruresis as men. The authors of *Shy Bladder Syndrome* write: "While social anxiety conditions are generally more prevalent among women, in terms of the clinical population, paruresis appears to be more common among men" (Soifer, et al., p. 12).

Men are far more inclined to seek help with paruresis than women. They sign up in greater numbers for IPA workshops and participate to a greater extent on the IPA's Internet Discussion Board. One explanation might simply reflect flaws and inadequacies in restroom design. Typically, men's bathrooms feature a lineup of adjacent urinals, often without partitions. A man receives no protection from the sounds, sights and even smells that accompany urination. The lack of an adequate number of stalls in men's restrooms may make it more difficult for men to deal with their paruresis. There may, however, be legitimate reasons for the under-representation of women.

o   Many women are unaware that they, too, are subject to paruresis while others may minimize its effect on their lives. The media has focused much of its attention on men who have "bashful bladder," sometimes disparagingly so. Articles about women and urination emphasize other female urinary dysfunctions, such as urinary incontinence or frequent urination, for which pharmaceutical companies have already found remedies. Some women suffer in silence, rationalizing their condition away ("*It's just something I have to put up with*"), and therefore do not seek help.

o The fact that more men enroll in IPA workshops may also reflect the wage disparity that separates the sexes. Many women deem it cost-prohibitive to travel to and attend a weekend workshop. Some women have expressed concerns about attending co-ed workshops because they fear men will dominate a mixed-discussion group.

o The lack of women's participation on the IPA Discussion Board may simply mean they are more inhibited about participating in open forums where they fear violation of their privacy. Some women, finding heavily male-oriented discussions, may think paruresis is a condition that affects only men and not bother to read further. Others are understandably reluctant to talk about personal issues with strangers, especially males; they prefer communicating directly with other women, either in person, by telephone, or by private e-mail exchange.

o More men than women may seek treatment because they feel their masculinity is being threatened. Some report feeling shame and humiliation if they can't "pee like a guy." Female paruretics, on the other hand, do not seem to feel the condition threatens their femininity.

Male Versus Female Bathroom Design and Behavior Patterns

Public bathrooms are uniquely designed for each sex, unless they are gender-neutral or family-friendly. Each gender demonstrates characteristic behavior patterns and attitudes. The chart on the next page illustrates some of these differences.

One major distinction is that while private stalls may be the backup option for some men in public restrooms, they are the **only** option available for women, unless they have learned to urinate in the wilds! A woman who cannot void in a private stall has only catheterization as a fall-back strategy, whether performed by herself or someone else.

	Men	**Women**
Standard toilet facilities in western-style public bathrooms	Urinals (often without dividers), private stalls (usually limited in number), troughs (occasionally).	Private stalls only (often not enough); lack of floor-to-ceiling privacy and soundproofing.
Enter the bathroom	Individually; may announce to a group they have to use the bathroom.	Individually; may ask a friend to accompany them; often enter in packs.
Bathroom behavior	"Get in, stand up, shut up, get out" (quickness and efficiency valued); seldom have eye contact; stare at feet; may converse with friends or business associates when entering but hardly ever with strangers.	Often linger to brush hair, apply make-up, change diapers, help disabled and elderly people, attend to personal needs; enjoy congregating and socializing; chat among each other while seated in an adjacent stall (humorously known as *"Gregarious Bladder Syndrome"*!).
Exit the bathroom	When men are done doing what they came in to do, they leave. If they are waiting on another guy to go back to wherever they came from, they wait outside.	Often will wait in the bathroom until they are all done, then leave together.
Encountering long lines	Sometimes (sports events, concerts, clubs).	Often. Can lead to paralyzing thought that *"someone is waiting for me."*
Noise level	Likely to be low, as silent as a library.	Can be high, depending on number of women in a public bathroom and decibel level.
Clothing	Release of a zipper.	Tends to be more complicated and time-consuming. Probably involves yanking something down around the knees – tugging, pulling, re-tucking.

Female bathroom behavior differs markedly from men's. Unlike men, women often enter public restrooms in packs, enjoying the social aspect and community-building that occurs when they congregate. Some converse between stalls or talk on their cell phones; others linger in restrooms while they apply make-up, perhaps change a baby's diaper, or attend to the needs of elderly family members. Some are accompanied by little children who can be disruptive when they share a stall with their mother. For a comical look at what goes on in women's restrooms, watch "The Ladies Room Monologues" at http://femalerestrooms.com.

For reasons of anatomy and culture, women take at least twice as long to complete a bathroom visit as men, according to studies. Dr. Clara Greed, a Professor of Inclusive Urban Planning and author of *Inclusive Urban Design,* offers several reasons why women face waits to use public toilets:

> …simply to check if one's period has actually started; if one's pants or tights are about to fall down, or if pregnancy…cystitis; to check on worries about vaginal discharge (or to check 'constantly' on one's 'whites' if one is using natural birth control to determine fertile days), and because they feel ill, are about to give birth or die; to pray; to cry and to get away, to think and be quiet; to escape from the city of man; and breast feeding (as a last resort) (Lowe, 2005).

Dr. Kathryn Anthony, a Professor of Architecture at the University of Illinois at Urbana-Champaign and a renowned expert on toilet design, reported the results from a research study by Edwards and McKie (1996) that analyzed myths surrounding why lines build around women's public toilets:

> They… point to both social and biological differences. Regarding social differences, women (in most western cultures) take more time in public restrooms because they must always come in direct contact with toilet surfaces unless they hover over a toilet. As young girls, they are taught to urinate sitting down in an enclosed cubicle and to use toilet paper and maybe a toilet seat cover. In contrast, men stand to urinate because they were taught to do so as boys and simply walk to an unenclosed urinal. Biologically, the female genitourinary system is internalized, whereas that of the male is externalized.

Furthermore, because about a quarter of all adult women are menstruating at any one time and a significant number of women may be pregnant, this adds to the length of time spent in the toilet as well as the number of toilet visits required in comparison to men (Anthony and Dufresne, 2007, p. 272).

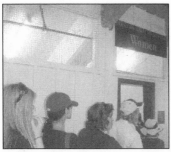

U.C. Berkeley football stadium

Photo by Carol Olmert

Paruretics, in general, don't like to feel rushed. Women face the possibility of long lines in often crowded bathrooms because there aren't enough stalls, an issue more commonly known as "Potty Parity." (Read Appendix 2 for a detailed discussion).

This may exacerbate the time pressure many already report feeling when they enter a restroom.

Still, common misperceptions exist between the genders. Many men think that women never have a problem with urinating in restrooms because they have the benefit of a stall and often go to the restroom in groups. Often women imagine that paruresis would not be something men would *ever* have because males are conditioned to learn to urinate in front of each other when they're kids and therefore never have problems.

Self-Catheterization Differs between the Sexes

Differences between male and female anatomy mean the self-catheterization process is not the same, and the risk of a urinary tract infection may be greater for women, as the table on the next page shows.

Given anatomical differences, the self-catheterization process is not the same for women as it is for men. It is highly recommended that women be taught by a knowledgeable health care practitioner, preferably a female, before attempting the process. Methods differ, but for practical purposes, it is useful to sit on or stand above a toilet, learning to identify the opening to the urethra by *"feel,"* then insert a catheter and allow the urine to drain into the toilet bowl. Detailed information about the self-catheterization process appears in "Survival Skills: Catheterization" in Chapter 8.

Catheters vary a great deal. They come in a large variety of sizes, materials, and types. In general, women are more likely to use catheters with smaller external diameters than those that men choose. For further information, see "Clean Intermittent Self Catheterization (CISC)" in Chapter 8.

	Men	*Women*
Anatomical differences	The male urethra is longer (varies from 17.5 to 20 cm.) than the female and runs the full length of the penis.	The female urethra is usually short (about 4 cm. long), making it easier for bacteria to gain entry to the bladder and multiply.
Identifying anatomical landmarks	Insertion of catheter through tip of penis normally by sight.	Insertion of catheter normally through feel. The female urethral orifice is located between the clitoris and the vagina and concealed.
Size of catheter	Probably one with a larger diameter, such as a 14 or 16 Fr*.	Probably one with a smaller diameter, such as a 12 Fr* or less.
Likelihood of developing urinary tract infections following catheterization (assuming use of clean intermittent techniques)	Less, but may increase after the age of 50. Most UTIs in adult males are complications of kidney or prostate infections.	At greater risk. One woman in five develops a UTI during her lifetime, according to statistics. Therefore women are encouraged to drink a lot of liquids and void often.

* The French (Fr) scale is used to measure catheter tubes;
1 FR equals one-third of a millimeter

Women are far more susceptible to urinary tract infections (UTIs or cystitis) than men, in general. One woman in five develops a UTI during her lifetime, according to statistics from the National Kidney and Urologic Diseases Information Clearinghouse ("National Kidney"). Even though antibiotics (e.g., Bactrim™, Septra™) can be prescribed for use as a preventative or treatment to alleviate UTI symptoms, many women prefer not to use a catheter because they fear the risk of infection.

In fact, in order to reduce the risk of urinary tract infections in the first place, women are advised to drink plenty of liquids, especially water, and to urinate frequently. Therein lies the *"Catch 22"* – a woman who is suffering from paruresis probably cannot and will not do that.

Chapter Three
Stall Tactics: How We Have Coped

As might be expected, female paruretics become very adept at developing avoidance behaviors and coping mechanisms to deal with their problem. Most of us have learned to accommodate to our condition, rather than seek treatment to recover from it.

The anticipation or reality of finding someone else in a bathroom can produce great anguish for many women plagued by paruresis. Some women will simply avoid entering any public restroom in which they even *sense* another may be present, instead running off to locate an isolated bathroom. Others adopt a strategy of "waiting it out" until everyone has disappeared; others will establish grand "schemes" or play "mind tricks" in order to cope.

At worst, many women will severely limit the amount of their fluid intake in order to avoid visiting public toilets. In one survey, 71% of 500 women said they often delay urinating because they are too busy, not near a bathroom or cannot find a sanitary bathroom ("Behind", 2002). Voluntary suppression of urination can lead to dehydration or further complications, such as urinary tract infections, bladder damage, or chronic kidney disease, according to the National Kidney and Urologic Diseases Information Clearinghouse ("Urinary Retention", n.d.) at http://kidney.niddk.nih.gov/index.htm

Let us, for a moment, take a look at examples of how some women deal with the presence of others in the bathroom. Be mindful of the psychological toll their behavior takes on their lives.

Making excuses

I make some excuse to be gone for a while and take off to a bathroom in another location (such as at the other end of the building, another floor, or another place altogether.) I basically warn friends that I will be gone 20 to 30 minutes and that gives me a safe window. That doesn't help in situations such as intermissions at plays, concerts, etc. so I just try to dehydrate myself – don't drink, especially coffee or alcohol, and I work out just before the outing and my body is on fluid conservation mode and I don't have to go. Otherwise I try to avoid situations where someone is waiting.

Unfortunately I practice avoidance behaviors in order to keep the feelings of anxiety away, and I've come to the realization that these days it's not that I CAN'T do certain things that I used to do (go camping, hiking, to the bars, travel, etc.) but that a lot of the joy has been taken out of these activities because of the anxiety, and that I usually don't WANT to do these things anymore. Within the parameters of my work and home life I feel very secure and comfortable, but it's only because I've curtailed my life to accommodate my paruresis.

Avoiding at any cost

Waiting it out

I'll be 36 next week and have had this problem for 26 years. All the faking and pretending just to go in and find someone in there and pretend you're only there to wash your hands or clean your glasses, or get an (invisible) stain off your skirt. I'm only a little bit better now that I'm a little older. I was in Disney World last year and did fine, since all the bathrooms are very large and noisy and basically, no one knows you're in there. But if it's a single bathroom, if someone is waiting, I can't go. My marriage broke up, and I believe in part because I wouldn't go on vacations or day trips. It's not the only reason, but I know it played a big part.

I have four levels of coping mechanisms: (1) "pretending" I'm combing my hair, applying lipstick or washing my hands until the person(s) leaves; (2) leaving the bathroom altogether to seek an empty facility, (3) returning to the original when I think everyone has left, or (4) if I really have to go badly and can't, then I catheterize myself.

Layers of coping mechanisms

Mind tricks, distraction, and grand schemes

If I am in a public stall, I will focus on something like a crack in the wall and hold my concentration on that.

I bring a crossword or word puzzle into a stall with me. Sometimes that helps me relax enough that I can begin to urinate.

I have done the fumbling around thing (like reaching into my purse for a tampon and using it) to make noise like there's a reason for me to be in there. On occasion, I have wadded up a bunch of toilet paper, dipped it in the obviously not pee-containing toilet water, and held it so that it drips the water back in, making it sound as though I'm peeing.

I take off a shoe and sock to feel the cold ground and get the flow started. Sometimes I try making funny faces to start peeing.

I stick my finger in the cold water of the toilet to start. Or I place my open palm very flatly against the tile or cold wall next to the toilet. These things always require some mental games before they work. I find myself thinking 'if only I could stick my finger in the cold water that would make things easier.' I have to gear up for it beforehand.

I create lists of things for myself to do right after I pee. I'll sit and think, 'Okay, pee and then you can pick that annoying thing up off the floor over there, and then wash your hands, and then blow your nose, and then put on some lip gloss, etc.' The list not only distracts me, but it makes the peeing part less important. Peeing is just something that needs to be done in a long list of tasks. Usually as soon as I pee though, I forget all about the crazy list.

I pretend to shoot myself in the head with my hand. I started that up when I was really depressed, and now I just do it when nobody is around and I'm frustrated.

When I'm truly in panic mode, I have often left the bathroom with bite marks on my hands. I don't realize that I'm doing it, but I bite my hands to distract myself and nearly draw blood!! This only happens when it's really bad and I'm shaking horribly. The worst part is that when I'm that terrified, there is NO WAY that I'm going to be able to pee!!!! I leave the bathroom all marked up, frustrated, and still with a full bladder.

Chapter Four
Now That You're Ready,
Hit the Road to Recovery

Are you ready to stop avoiding restrooms? Here are six initial steps you can take.

1. If you suspect you might have paruresis, start by ruling out the possibility you have a bona fide physical disorder and consult with a health care professional. Since few of these professionals are familiar with paruresis, I recommend you bring along with you some descriptive material that explains the condition. Sometimes what appears to be paruresis may actually be a physiological condition. For instance, it may be Neurogenic Bladder, a dysfunction of the bladder due a malfunction of the autonomic nerves that control bladder function—or another bladder disorder.

The American Urological Association has published an excellent article on paruresis, which can be found in Appendix 4 or at http://www.urologyhealth.org/.

2. Absorb all the introductory information about paruresis on the IPA Home Page at www.paruresis.org. Educate yourself about paruresis. Understand the effects of adrenaline, anxiety, and avoidance. Learn the difference between primary paruresis (the physical symptom, locking up) and secondary paruresis (the emotional and behavioral reactions to having difficulty urinating around others – guilt, anxiety, shame, embarrassment, helplessness, etc.). Discover you are not alone! Understand that, at least in respect to paruresis, there are more commonalities than differences between women and men.

3. Read educational materials. It is much easier to get started on a recovery program when you have read some of the following materials and understand why certain things are encouraged and others are discouraged. Books by the following authors and titles are recommended:

o Dr. Steven Soifer's pioneering book, *Shy Bladder Syndrome: Your Step-by-Step Guide to Overcoming Paruresis.* Considered the definitive book on the subject, it is available from the IPA Book Store at www.paruresis.org or through Amazon.com (www.amazon.com). (Dr. Soifer is the IPA co-founder and CEO.)

o Dr. Howard Liebgold's booklets and tapes entitled *Curing Phobias, Shyness & Obsessive Compulsive Disorders* (also referred to as "Phobease") offer practical advice in treating social anxiety conditions such as paruresis. He also teaches classes and is a member of the IPA Advisory Board. Go to www.angelnet.com/fear.html.

o Dr. Christopher McCullough's book, *Free to Pee: A Self-Help Guide for Men with Paruresis,* is also available from the IPA Store at www.paruresis.org. While geared toward the male audience, this book provides useful information on paruresis and how to deal with it. In essence, you learn how to be comfortable being anxious. Visit www.paruresis.org/notes_on_AP.htm.

o Self-help books that use Cognitive-Behavioral Therapy as the foundation are valuable resources. Among them:

  • *Guide to Rational Living* by Dr. Albert Ellis.

  • *Anxiety Disorders and Phobias: A Cognitive Perspective* by Dr. Aaron T. Beck.

  • *Brain Lock (Free Yourself from Obsessive-Compulsive Behavior)* – and other titles – by Dr. Jeffrey Schwartz.

  • Several books on anxiety and phobias by Dr. Edmund J. Bourne.

o Books that describe and offer insights into biologically and emotionally more sensitive people, such as Dr. Elaine Aron's *The Highly Sensitive Person* and Dr. Ted Zeff's *The Highly Sensitive Person's Survival Guide.*

A more complete list of books appears on the IPA website (www.paruresis.org/books.htm).

4. Log on and register in order to read the posts on the IPA Talk Forums – an Internet Discussion Board – at http://paruresis.org/phpBB3/ (another useful website is www.paruretic.com). Remember: you can use an alias when registering – you need not use your real name if you have any privacy issues. YOU WILL LEARN A LOT!!! If nothing else, you will discover you are not the only person in the world who suffers from this condition and also begin to develop empathy for yourself and others. When you are comfortable, either respond to a post or submit one of your own. Continue to be an active participant on the Board, where you will find an immediate connection to fellow paruretics.

5. Read about issues unique to female paruretics on the IPA website.

A separate section, "Women's Resources," is available on the Home Page at www.paruresis.org/womens_resources.htm. Here you will find information that is exclusively focused on female paruretic issues; it also includes the publication of some of the previous electronic newsletters I have authored for women only.

6. Join and become active in the IPA's Women-Only forum.

Equally important, an IPA Discussion Board, entitled "Women Only," was created in 2006. A private and "hidden" forum, it is open only to and moderated by women. In order to participate, follow these instructions:

o Log on to the IPA website (www.paruresis.org).

o First register as a user (with an alias, if you wish), then:

o Write to womensforum@paruresis.org. In the subject field, include the words "new member." Tell us you would like to subscribe and remember to include your user name.

o We will then add your name to our user group and notify you when we have done so.

o You will then have access and can begin to communicate solely with other women.

Chapter Five
Why Can't I Be Normal, Like All the Others?

Many of us, in our desire for perfection and need to "fit in," continually berate ourselves for our difficulties in not being able to urinate like everyone else. This chapter addresses some of these concerns, challenges your thinking about normalcy, and introduces you to ways in which you can combat your negative self-talk.

Challenge your thinking: What is "normal"?

"Why can't I just be normal, like all the others?" you may ask yourself.

Well, the truth is, not only are you normal, but quite likely you are a special woman with heightened sensitivities and sensibilities. If you're anything like me, you may be a woman with an ultra-sensitive nervous system. I prefer to think of us as being more sensitized than others, and our symptoms just happen to hit us around our bladders.

Writing in her best-selling book, *The Highly Sensitive Person: How to Thrive When the World Overwhelms You*, Dr. Elaine N. Aron describes some of the characteristics of this type of individual:

> ...tends to be easily overwhelmed when in a highly stimulating environment for too long... is affected by other people's moods... picks up on the subtleties in their surroundings that others miss...may be easily startled and need to withdraw during busy times to a private, quiet place...and gets nervous or shaky if someone is observing them or competing with them (Aron, 1996).

Highly sensitive people – or HSPs, as Aron calls the estimated 15% to 20% of the population who possess this trait – have a low threshold for excessive stimulation (noisy crowds, bright lights, etc.) and a heightened awareness to everything in their environment. Furthermore, according to Aron, they were probably born this way. Their intense arousal to stimuli that goes unobserved by others (sounds, sights, physical sensations) isn't due to a personality flaw in their makeup but to the way their brain functions and the way it processes information.

The trait of high sensitivity is completely "normal," not a psychological disorder in need of repair. Many of us HSPs have grown up in a culture which doesn't appreciate sensitivity and been negatively impacted by some stereotypes others hold of us. Often we're branded as being shy, worry-warts, slow, introverted, over-emotional, aloof, or neurotic, even by some professionals. Aron's research is a welcome effort to show the world that "not being the same as the societal ideal" does NOT necessarily have to be labeled as a pathology. Highly sensitive people, she contends, should not try to become less sensitive but rejoice in the special gifts that being highly sensitive brings, such as keener intuition, enhanced perceptivity, and the ability to sense danger and trouble sooner than most.

Appreciate who you are; treasure your uniqueness

While Dr. Aron's study appears grounded in solid research and persuasive scientific explanations, as well as in her personal experiences and those of numerous subjects she interviewed, the IPA lacks hard data to suggest that paruretics truly are more sensitive than non-paruretics.

However, in my experience, many of us paruretics tend to be compassionate, good, fair, conscientious, and intelligent people whose qualities should be celebrated, not berated.

In a society that values the characteristics of ambition, competition, goal orientation, extroversion, and time urgency, those of us with sensitive nervous systems are more easily overwhelmed by intense levels of stimulation. We can learn new routines that may help us disconnect from the fast-paced world in which we live, including exercising our bodies (gentle stretching, yoga postures or light calisthenics), calming our minds (through meditation and deep breathing exercises), and living more contemplative lives. Some of these techniques are further described in the "Breathing, Breath Holding, and Relaxation Techniques" section in Chapter 9.

Many of us paruretics tend to be extremely polite people who don't want to offend or inconvenience others, or who put others' feelings above their own. In fact, part of your recovery program will involve learning to and tolerating putting yourself first, not last. Once you accept that you are just as important as the next person, you are more than halfway toward your recovery.

I know that, for myself, it has taken me years to fully understand, accept and appreciate my sensitive nervous system, as well as the qualities that make me different from others in a special way.

Accept yourself and embrace your humanity

First of all, it's not your fault that you are paruretic. You did nothing to create your symptoms. So accept yourself and forgive yourself for what you consider to be an "imperfection." Feel good about who you are.

Acceptance is one of the most important things that can advance your recovery. I accept myself as being nervous at times. I accept myself and ask for help and understanding. I'm not perfect. I am who I am, a nice, empathetic woman with some anxiety.

Many of us tend to expect perfection of ourselves. We may view the process of urinating as one which "is supposed to happen in a certain way." A lot of us are concerned with the time we take, the strength of our stream, the amount we pass, etc. As paruretics, we find it hard to "go with the flow" (pun intended!) and take each attempt for what it is.

It is self-defeating to compare yourself to others and judge yourself inferior

Urination is not a competition in which you're trying to be the best or "perfect," nor is it a performance test. It is simply a necessary body function we all need to do. How you do it does not reflect on your worth. There is no requirement that you be fast enough, loud enough, or "perfect" enough.

Yes, there will always be someone in the next stall who urinates without hesitation or who has a nice strong stream. Accept that. Accept that the inability to void is okay and is part of the recovery process. The pursuit of perfection and the failure to achieve it will only set you up for frustration and disappointment – in this and every aspect of your life.

Remember, we all have strengths and weaknesses. It is the using of our strengths to help others when they may be weak that makes for a loving and compassionate world. So acknowledge, appreciate, and develop your own special talents, recognizing that the ability to urinate "on demand" may not be one of them.

Chapter Six
Exploring Fears and Concerns

While many of us may never know what event, circumstance or experience first triggered our paruresis, we realize that our condition has taken on a life of its own that often disrupts our ability to function. Knowing the etiology will not help you recover.

Paruresis, as we've learned, is a social anxiety that thrives on secrecy, shame and avoidance. We paruretics perceive restrooms or the presence of others in them as a threat – whether on a conscious or subconscious level – which may result in the physical inability to urinate.

When you enter a restroom, you may experience physical symptoms of anxiety, such as nausea, dizziness, heart palpitations, trembling, tense muscles, and sweating. For some, the anxiety will intensify into a panic attack. These symptoms of anxiety often lead to further embarrassment for the person with paruresis.

Some sufferers with less pronounced physical symptoms may still feel very self-conscious and afraid.

Given that those with social anxiety experience marked mental and physical anxiety, they tend to avoid the feared social situations and in severe cases may therefore be very socially isolated.

Common triggers

Some common psychological triggers that cause our brains to lock up when urinating include proximity to others, invasion of personal space, presence of strangers, lack of visual or auditory privacy, sensitivity to noise, and temporary psychological states, especially anxiety, anger, and fear, that can interfere with urination.

The next section explores in greater depth some of the fears and concerns that female paruretics have and presents some suggestions for ways to deal with them.

o Fear of telling others.

o Fear of taking too long.

o The common fears – being seen, being heard, being next to someone, personal space invasion.

o The root of the problem – caring too much about what others think.

Telling Others about Our Shy Bladders

How and when to disclose paruresis to others

As we've discovered, paruresis is considered one form of a specific social anxiety. However, it differs from other kinds, such as the fear of speaking in public or writing, eating or drinking in front of others, to the extent it is less known about, socially "acceptable" (in our minds), and therefore harder to disclose. Unlike some of those other feared social situations that can perhaps be more easily avoided or managed, our fear of bathrooms can be debilitating emotionally and potentially harmful to our bodies.

The knowledge alone that there are others like you and me out there – perhaps as many as 7% of the population – may make it easier for you to reveal your condition to others.

Telling others in our lives

Let's face it. The disclosure of personal information about yourself to another – the admission of what you perceive as a character "flaw" or "defect" – can be challenging, if not traumatic. It is especially difficult for young adults who are trying to "fit in" and are unsure of themselves around others. We often expect perfection of ourselves and others, so we allow our fears to get in the way of sharing our vulnerabilities with each other. Feeling ashamed of our condition, which we did nothing to create in the first place, we often go to extraordinary lengths to keep it a secret from others.

Although paruresis responds readily to treatment, many people remain undiagnosed or misdiagnosed, in part because they are embarrassed to admit their condition.

Here are some examples of common fears that prevent us from telling.

No one will really understand

I've told one teenage friend, my whole family, one other grown-up friend, (and will no doubt tell several more when the moment strikes). The teenage friend is nice about it, understands the single-stall use – but not completely. It's hard for it to sink in that 'no, no, no, even if you're waiting quietly outside for me, it doesn't help and heightens my fear,' or that 'no, if you come in and shout for me, it doesn't make me feel any safer, in fact worse!', which is frustrating.

If I tell my close women friends, I'm afraid they will say, "Oh, that happens to me sometimes, too," but I know that for these people they can pee pretty much anywhere any time and what they liken shy bladder to is not being able to pee immediately. They miss the distinction that I could sit there until the cows came home and I wasn't going to be able to pee with someone in the room.

I'm afraid of being laughed at if I tell someone

I've been thinking lately about telling a good friend of mine. We have been close friends since 5th grade. We are now 27 years old. One fear that I have is that she would tell other people, and they would laugh behind my back. I know that sounds really bad, like I don't trust her, but I just feel like such a weirdo with this problem.

Now they'll be paying more attention to me

It is still hard for me to share my paruresis with additional friends and family members. I feel like once they know, they will be paying attention to me in future situations.

My life experiences have taught me that almost everyone has her or his share of problems, fears, and concerns, though they may be unable to admit them to themselves and/or unwilling to let others know about them. Many people cannot let others see their flaws because they fear loss of acceptance, disapproval, or rejection. Some of them may even have urinary hesitancy problems too – they simply do not make a big deal out of them.

Challenge your thinking: What happens if you tell?

What if you were to change your thinking for a moment? Can you imagine the possibility of creating a stronger bond – fostering intimacy – with the person you tell? Might your disclosure of "weakness" give someone else the permission they need to reveal something highly personal about themselves? How liberating that can be for each of us!

Thinking negatively or irrationally, we expect the worst case scenario to result if we open up to others. In our tendency to catastrophize, we fail to ask ourselves some important questions:

o What is my worst fear – ridicule? disapproval? rejection? abandonment?

o Can I live with that? Do I really want or need to have someone in my life who does not at least empathize with my situation?

o How would I respond if someone told me a deep, dark "secret"?

Now consider the best case scenario. Once you tell friends and family members about your paruresis, you'll find that they will be more understanding, and you'll be less nervous around them when the need arises to use a restroom. That alone may reduce anxiety and make it easier to urinate. Observe that most people are supportive and don't view paruresis in the same catastrophic or shameful way that you do. This will help you begin to see that a lot of the shame and guilt you feel don't exist in others; it is self-generated as a consequence of the affliction.

Be selective, but be open

o Use discrimination when choosing with whom to share your condition. If you think the other person will ridicule, discount or judge you harshly, it's best not to share the information.

o Telling trusted and non-judgmental individuals, close friends, and family members is a good way to begin. For teenagers, who might find that their schoolmates can be viciously cruel, I would recommend speaking to a school counselor or nurse about how to address this problem. People you don't feel would be likely to support you are not good allies in helping you with your goal of recovery. People in the workplace may not be a good choice if you feel sharing the information might be used against you in any way or make you feel too vulnerable.

o Prepare well in advance so that you are likely to feel more comfortable, self-confident, and calm during and after the disclosure. Because paruresis is a relatively less known condition than, say, claustrophobia or fear of heights, know that you are going to have to educate your listener.

o Explain paruresis and its effects on your life in a clear, simple, almost nonchalant way (only you can determine how much detail to go into). Encourage discussion afterwards.

o If you encounter a negative or insensitive response from a person, try not to let it affect you. People who are ignorant or condescending toward those with paruresis probably lack empathy and the inability to help and support others. See it as their problem, not yours. There are a small number of people like that you may encounter, and the best course is to avoid them. By sharing your paruresis with those you trust, you will find supportive help. The benefits you will gain from reaching out to the good people in your lives far outweigh the risks.

o Remember, it is not necessary to tell everyone, and it gets much easier over time.

Experiences of women who have told others

Just telling people about my condition works well for me

Just 'tell' people that you have difficulty urinating and it takes you a while. You don't need to explain why; they will just think you have a medical problem, which is true and no reason to be ashamed. I've used this method before and it works. It takes the time pressure off of you and in this day and age of political correctness, they probably won't dig deeper.

It's much easier to be honest and direct

Most of my close friends know about this, and several even know about the catheters. I could have never told anyone years ago, but I've decided it's been easier to be honest because sometimes I would appear sneaky and suspicious – running to a faraway bathroom, in there forever when I was green at self-cathing, not paying attention and acting fishy and uptight because I'm plotting how to "move the party" away from the bathroom in a small place, etc. Now I can tell most of my friends, "I gotta pee. I'm gonna turn the water on. Don't listen!"

I guess telling my oldest and closest friends was the most interesting. I could finally tell them why for all these years I have always suddenly disappeared after a day out and why I didn't like staying over. They told me they could finally understand why I would be so odd at times! That was the worst bit: to discover that my "odd" way had been noticed and there was me trying very hard to convince myself nobody would notice! Anyway, it has meant that when I go out with them now if I'm really having trouble I can tell them, and I can't tell you how wonderful that is because it really does make life so much better.

One uses the analogy of "coming out" (as a lesbian) to friends and family

I came out as a lesbian when I was 16 (I'm 46 now), and I do feel that revealing one's sexual orientation is very similar to revealing one's paruresis. Not that these are the same things, but the feelings can be similar. There are folks who just won't understand you, others who might minimize things (what's the big deal?), and others who will accept and support you.

Coming out with the paruresis thing was much more charged for me. I feel no shame with respect to my sexuality, but I still feel some shame about this. Although my shame level is way reduced, it still exists. I think what we think in our own heads about how others will react is usually worse than what really happens.

One thing that has helped me in overcoming paruresis is to get out of my own head – *nobody cares* about me peeing. *Nobody* cares if I take an hour to start or if I start and stop. *Nobody* cares anything about me while I'm peeing or waiting to pee. This problem is way bigger to us than to anyone else. We major in it. I do believe this now, but it took time to sink in.

The first time is the hardest

I found it very difficult to 'come out' about having paruresis. I figured I finally had to break the silence and shame around it and decided to trust my very good friend. I was nervous telling her. I think I said something along the lines of 'I have trouble peeing in public bathrooms.' She asked some questions and was supportive and didn't minimize the issue at all. I explained that I felt most comfortable in a private lockable single-seater and that the most difficult place was a two-seater (like at work).

This friend is a long time one (10ish years), and over the years we have grown to trust each other, and even though I know she wouldn't react badly, I still had trouble and was very nervous disclosing this information. That's how large the shame was for me.

I think the first time you reveal this information is the hardest. And then when you realize that most people will be supportive and won't run for the hills or laugh at us until they wet their pants (or whatever reaction you fear the most) it takes some of the magnitude out of the demon.

It wasn't such a big deal

One of the close female friends I told was expecting it to be a much bigger 'deal' based on my nervousness in the conversation. She said she felt sorry for me that I had suffered from this for so long. She said it must be horrible and stressful. The other female friend I told was very uncomfortable in the conversation. I think she knew it was a huge ordeal for me, and she just didn't know what to say. She is usually an advisor, and I think this was a subject she just didn't know anything about.

I've had paruresis for about 40 years. I'm 46 years old. At first it was very difficult to tell people. I started with my mother and husband. Now I talk about it much more openly, and that seems to have taken some of the fear away and the power shy bladder carries over me quite a bit. Sometimes I say to friends that I have problems peeing in public restrooms and sometimes other places. I might also add that it's a more common problem than I realized, but most of the people I know who have it are men. I've told friends I'm having a little trouble with the bathroom in this restaurant; I'm going to step outside and see if there is something else nearby (like a Subway) that I can use before we go to the movies. This tactic has helped me not stress as much and also helped me make plans that before I wouldn't have made.

Time Pressures – "Someone Is Waiting for Me"

Female paruretics think that others think they take too long

Women's bathrooms tend to be crowded, with lines often forming to use too few stalls. This situation can cause great distress for the female paruretic as she has to contend with time pressure, or the paralyzing thought that "someone is waiting for me to finish."

This issue of "Potty Parity" – the huge disparity that exists between the time men and women wait to use restroom facilities in public places – has commanded a lot of media attention and is being addressed at various levels. As of 2006, at least 21 states and a number of municipalities have laws requiring doubling, tripling and even quadrupling the ratio of women's-to-men's toilets in public buildings. (For more about this subject, see the "Gender Equity in Bathrooms" section in Appendix 2).

But maybe someone – a friend, colleague, or acquaintance – really is waiting for you to finish up your business so you can walk out together. Then what?

Vicious circle

What happens when I think that people think that I am taking too long in the bathroom – how the vicious circle begins:

My paruresis is definitely triggered in part by any thoughts that somebody is waiting for me. It's too much pressure. It's not so much that I feel I don't deserve my time in the bathroom; I just get nervous that I won't be able to do it, and then I'm not able to, and then I think people are thinking I'm taking too long, and the more I think that, the more I can't do it, and what a vicious cycle it becomes.

I am most troubled by perceived 'time pressures,', e.g., I have to plan very carefully to urinate before someone arrives to visit me at home, as I often cannot go when people are there.

Handling time pressure when someone is waiting

In his best-selling book, *Future Shock*, published in 1970, Alvin Toffler was one of the first to write about the symptoms of this condition. He described future shock as "the shattering stress and disorientation that we induce in individuals by subjecting them to too much change in too short a time (Toffler, 1970, p.2). One of the ideas Toffler proposed was that people could become overwhelmed and disoriented with the onslaught of new information, as well as the speed-up of daily life.

Today we live in a highly competitive, technological, media- and consumer-driven culture. Our society values the ability to handle high levels of stimulation over the ability to reflect, to multi-task rather than focus our complete attention on any one activity.

Over-stimulation in our society has increased at an alarming rate. Inarguably, many people have adopted the prevailing modern notion that faster is better and that everything is a race against the clock.

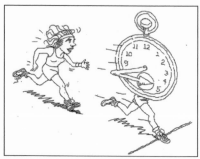

Illustration by Ericka Hamburg

erickahamburg.com; used with permission

We have become a sped-up society. Technological advances have expanded the business day. Leisure time has shrunk. Speed dating has become common. On weekends, business people in swimsuits walk on beaches with cellular phones stuck to their ears, planning the next morning's meetings.

Laptop computers find their way on vacations. The family icons of today are working couples picking up their children on their way home to dinners prepared by caterers, fast food chefs, or manufacturers of microwavable dishes. Grieving time has shrunk. The divorce rate hovers near its highest in history. The concept of job security seems outmoded. There is no time to pick up the pieces. "Just snap out of it," one friend tells another.

For some women, feeling pressured about time extends to other realms of their life beyond bathrooms. One contributor to the IPA Women's Forum wrote: *"I know that time-waiting issues are critical for me. I feel them even when I'm using a copy machine and a couple of people are waiting in line in back of me. I don't know where I learned to subordinate my right to take my time doing a task to others, but it is clear that somewhere along the line I learned precisely that."*

Perhaps to some degree we can "blame" the socialization process on the ways in which women are taught – sometimes subtly and sometimes not – to be polite. Think about some of the admonitions that come from well-meaning parents, grandparents, aunts, uncles, and innumerable teachers: "Stand up and let the lady *(obviously written by a man!)* take the seat on the bus." "Let that old man go ahead of you." "Hurry up, you're taking up *their* time."

Challenge your thinking:
Is everyone really waiting for you to use a stall?

As a paruretic, you probably think to yourself, "Someone or everyone is waiting for me to use my stall, and I must hurry." You probably have an internal clock in your head that tells you that you're taking too long – one minute in a stall can seem like an eternity. A few seconds of delayed onset seems like you are taking forever.

I encourage you to challenge your theories and assumptions.

Your assignment is to produce evidence that combats your thoughts. Here are some approaches:

o   Take a closer look at your own personal experience. If you obsess that "everyone is watching you use the stall," stop and ask yourself whether anyone really has ever noticed or verbalized some criticism of you when doing so.

o   Prove to yourself that no one is watching, listening, or paying attention to you. Deliberately sit on a toilet seat – with no urge or intention of urinating. Just sit there determined not to do anything and feeling in charge of the time, then leaving and feeling okay about it. Begin with three minutes and increase your time to 15 minutes until you become very adept. *Notice if anyone says anything to you* or even notices you. They are probably thinking about other things or preoccupied with themselves. ("What am I going to have for lunch today?")

And, even if someone noticed or said something derogatory, would that really be a catastrophe? Yes, you would probably feel embarrassed and maybe even ashamed, but would that be the end of the world, or would these just be feelings that have a beginning, middle, and an end? (Robbins, March 5, 2006).

This is an example of a type of exposure exercise that is further described in the "Treatment of Paruresis" (Chapter 9).

Learn tools to help you relax and reduce stress

The methods by which you can better cope with time pressure are practical and suit many situations, not just feeling hurried in a bathroom. By learning and practicing these techniques, you can greatly decrease the intensity of your anxiety and reduce the frequency of the intense feelings.

You can create new daily routines that:

o Exercise your body (gentle stretching, yoga postures or light calisthenics).

o Calm your mind in order to disengage from a stressful environment (through meditation, deep breathing exercises, muscle relaxation positive imagery, and other means of relaxation).

o Make sure you allow for sufficient private downtime.

o Help you learn to live a more contemplative life.

For further discussion on such routines and their benefits, see the "Breathing, Breath-Holding, and Relaxation Techniques" section in Chapter 9.

In addition, you may want to try individual or group counseling or attend a stress reduction class.

These are some of the techniques I and others have employed in order to reduce stress in our lives:

o Listen to a relaxation CD or classical and soothing music.

o Take long, deep breaths.

o Practice meditation techniques.

o Visualize a graphical image that is "pleasant or soothing" to you, such as a nature scene.

> *Change your thoughts and you change your world.*
>
> Norman Vincent Peale
> Clergyman (1898–1993)

o Talk more slowly.

o Spend time in silence while in the presence of family and friends.

o Create restorative environments.

o Avoid trying to do two or three or more things at a time.

o Give up trying to be perfect and feeling like you must do everything.

o Avoid people who are "stress carriers."

o Organize your work; set priorities.

o Limit caffeine and alcohol intake.

o Maintain your health with good nutrition, sleep and rest.

o Get regular exercise.

o Take a walk in nature.

o When stressed, ask yourself "Is this really important?" and "Will this even matter to me next year, next month, or next week?"

Encountering Others in Bathrooms – Being Seen, Heard, or Too Close to Others

As noted earlier, women spend more time in restrooms than men because of anatomical, biological, and cultural differences. Their behavior in bathrooms is also far different because they often:

o Enter the restroom in packs.

o Chat in front of and across stalls or in the waiting area.

o Apply make-up or other cosmetics.

o Bring a young child or maybe an older person into a stall.

The issue:
Finding others in bathrooms while you are desperate to be alone (and will seek any means to do so)

The anticipation or reality of finding someone else in a bathroom can produce great anguish for many female paruretics.

As we've seen in the previous chapter on coping strategies of female paruretics, each of us manages differently – through avoidance, waiting it out, or developing simple or elaborate "mind games" or distraction techniques.

The most common concerns seem to be: "I Might Be Seen," "I Might Be Heard," "I Might Be Sensed" or "Someone Is Close to Me" (both *physically* – the relative closeness of others in or near the restroom – and *psychologically*, involving the need for privacy for self).

Does this sound like you? Do you fear that:

o Everyone's attention is focused on you?

o You will make mistakes and everyone will notice?

o Everyone else is more capable than you in the same situation?

o You are being judged by others?

o You will embarrass or humiliate yourself in front of others?

Writes one woman:

It depends on how much I think the other person(s) is NOT paying any attention to me. I sometimes think people who are very quiet and sit for minutes at a time are 'listening' to what I'm doing. Nevertheless, for many years, I could not urinate, even while alone, if I had even the slightest idea that someone might come into the bathroom.

Writes another:

My problem has involved every angle I can think of. But time pressure, someone hearing, stalls where you can see through the doors and can see the person's feet next to you, even getting too uptight about something, that I have had to catheterize myself while alone at home. Prior to catheters, I have sat on many toilets, red in the face with anger and tears at the impossibility of relieving myself.

The Root of the Problem –
Caring Too Much What Others May Think

Remember, paruresis is a type of social anxiety so that, for most, other people are the cause of anxiety. Social anxiety creates in us the feeling that we are being watched and judged by others, even if sometimes rationally we know that this is not the case.

Some of us profess not to care about what others are thinking. They disavow being plagued by WOPT (What Other People Think).

One young lady writes:

> I am such a confident person, not shy at all, Valedictorian of my class, four-time class President, and in general I sincerely do not mind what people think of me. I've never been afraid to go against the crowd. But when it comes to the bathroom... It's just so odd.
>
> During a trip with my classmates, I suffered through several failed attempts in the restroom. What agony it is, sitting in there, in that little stall at a rest stop, bladder full, the urge to pee intense, mind coaxing and trying to relax, but body utterly refusing! What agony it is, sitting in there for several minutes, trying every little mind trick I know, and being ALMOST on the VERGE of it starting to flow...and having it be a no-go. Defeat, utter defeat. On occasions like that I walk out of the bathroom feeling like a lawyer who's fought the fight of his life, only to lose his innocent man to a death sentence. Not to mention the loneliest chump on earth.

Another says:

> I have a pretty healthy self esteem, and couldn't care less what anybody thinks of me, especially strangers. I could never figure this one out myself. Why can't I go if I don't care what this other person, dilly-dallying around in a one or two "seater" bathroom, thinks of me just sitting there and not going, or whatever? I guess, subconsciously, I must worry about it, but then I can't figure out why I'd be worrying about such a silly thing.

The option:
Change your thinking about bathrooms and the people in them and you will begin to change your life

As I mentioned earlier, the best place to initiate a change in your thinking is to stop viewing urination in public or private as a performance test. It is simply a necessary body function we all do. It doesn't matter how you do it, how fast or strong your urine stream is, or whether the act of expelling urine is 100% "*perfect.*"

> ## What other people think about me is not my business.
>
> Michael J. Fox
> In *Lucky Man* – a memoir
> Actor (1961 -)

Many women have triumphed over paruresis by taking the time to analyze and confront their irrational thought patterns about women in bathrooms. They have transcended their fears by replacing their distorted thought patterns with more accurate statements. They have learned to claim their entitlement to remain in a toilet stall for as long as they want or need.

Carl Robbins, IPA co-founder and Director of the Training, Anxiety and Stress Disorders Institute of Maryland, suggests ways you can benefit from examining your fears of WOPT.

Example: I think people might think strange things of me. ('That girl... she coughs while in the bathroom! What is she thinking?!')

Ask yourself some of the following questions:

1. How good are you at mind-reading?
2. How do you know that other people are paying attention to what *you* are doing in the restroom?
3. What else might they think if you made noise (coughed) besides "What is she thinking?"
4. Would it really be a *catastrophe* if people thought negative things about you?
5. What price are you willing to pay to eliminate the *possibility* that someone might find out you have paruresis? Is it worth it?

Experiment: Ask 50 people who do not have paruresis what they notice when they enter a bathroom. You will probably find that almost all are somewhere else mentally, and, in fact, there is pressure on people not to notice what you are doing. As Alexander Kira, author of the classic, *The Bathroom,* pointed out, "the rules of social conduct ...ensure that no one will pay very close attention, either to one's person or one's activities" (Kira, p. 207). The source of embarrassment, then, would be "Oh, I am paying attention to someone else's urine stream, what's wrong with me?" (Robbins, May 28, 2007).

You are likely to conclude that:

o Your fears about what others think are largely unfounded. Most of the people you know don't really think about you much at all. They probably are too busy thinking about themselves and their own lives to be making conclusions about yours.

o Even if others do think about you from time to time, you may misinterpret what they might be thinking and assume it's something negative.

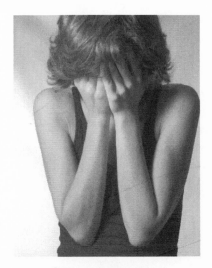

© Photo by gumibaya

Image from BigStockPhoto.com

We may be concerned about what others think of us because we have learned to be highly critical of others. Also, we are often highly critical of ourselves. But just because we are highly critical doesn't mean that others are, too. They may not only be caught up in their own world, but when they do think about us, they are a lot kinder to us than we are to ourselves.

Now, let's say someone does notice that you have a weak stream, etc. As Carl Robbins further elucidates, s/he would probably conclude "I'm glad that's not me" or "I feel sorry for that person."

Please understand that this is not about NOT CARING what other people think. Sure, everyone likes to be admired, respected, and thought well of. The question is what ELSE do you care about besides how you appear to others? Might there be a higher priority than impression management when you attempt to urinate (e.g., taking whatever time you need to empty your bladder so that you can get on with your life?) (Robbins, November 22, 2006).

If you are afraid of being evaluated or judged, ask yourself whether this is reasonable. Try and realize that you can only do your best and that will have to be good enough. If you get criticized (highly unlikely), well, you are only human. And you will most likely find the only one being critical of you is *you*!

The technique for changing thinking patterns to help overcome your fears, *Cognitive Restructuring*, is fully described in the "Treatment of Paruresis" section in Chapter 9.

Chapter Seven
Practical Do's and Don'ts

While I believe that Cognitive-Behavior Therapy offers the greatest promise for recovery in the long term, I am also a strong proponent of the "whatever works" method in the short term. Toward that end, I have included some tools and techniques that might help you to urinate in various situations.

In this chapter, you will find some practical steps you can take to maximize your chances of urinating when you're concerned about noise (too much or too little) in a bathroom, traveling (by airplane, train, boat, or car), and using restrooms in foreign countries.

Noise in the Bathroom

The issue:
Many female paruretics are keenly sensitive to the sounds they or others make in a bathroom

Even if the spacing of toilets in a public restroom is sufficient to use the facility, the fear of producing sounds or hearing those of others may prevent you from being able to urinate in a public bathroom.

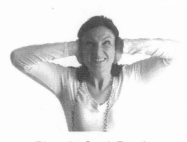

Some women are intolerant of noise that others make in the bathroom (chatting, conversations with each other or with you).

Photo by Sarah Brooke

sarahbrookephotography.co.uk/
Reprinted with permission

Suggestions

o Challenge your thinking: How do noises make you nervous?

o The iPod solution: How to reduce or increase the sound level in a bathroom.

o New inventions and technologies that may help.

o Create soundproof stalls.

Noise affects female paruretics in different ways. What may be a disturbing noise for one person may be a pleasant sound for someone else. Some women seem ultra-sensitive to noise, to the possibility of being "heard" while urinating, or to the presence of external or ambient noise, such as from fans, hand dryers, or background music, in the restroom. Other women are particularly sensitive to the noise that others in the bathroom may create, either as a result of conversations or even the unwrapping of a tampon in an adjacent stall.

Some women claim it is always impossible for them to urinate in a quiet bathroom. On the other hand, others think the absence of noise creates a relaxing environment that allows them to urinate, so they prefer very quiet bathrooms.

Sounds shut her down

> If I hear any sound – music playing, fans blowing, toilets flushing, anyone talking – I cannot relax enough to pee.

She heads to the farthest stall

> One of the things that really shuts me down is going into one of those gigantic rest rooms like they have at large movie theaters. Because I prefer it to be real quiet, I find a stall way off in the corner.

Thumbs down on automatic flushes

> Those new automatic flush toilets drive me crazy because I'm startled by the noise they make and disruption they cause.

Challenge your thinking: How noises make you nervous

Consider the following thought, "*noises make me anxious*." Understand that noise is the activating event. Then there is the consequence of that – you experience anxiety or, in the worst case, the inability to urinate, and then there may be a behavioral consequence, which is to either avoid or flee. In between the activating event and the consequence is a belief or a thought that actually mediates how the activating event becomes the anxiety-producing consequence. It is at this point that you ask yourself, "How do noises create anxiety for me?"

Examine a second thought, *"I can hear them, so they can hear me."* Now think that one through. Say to yourself, *"and then"*? What does it mean if they hear you? Will they make fun of you? So what? And how did you reach that conclusion in the first place?

Create a thought journal. Write down your beliefs or thoughts – and begin to challenge them. Put a lot of detail into it. Over time, when you re-read your entries, you will begin to note a pattern of progress.

The iPOD solution:
Changing bathroom sound levels

For those women who are bothered by sounds in bathrooms, devices are available that can mitigate noise. You can:

- o Bring a CD or MP3 player with headphones into a stall. Use it to play soothing music or listen to a relaxation exercise.

- o Buy a white noise machine to help drown out startling noises by emitting a steady soothing sound.

- o Wear earmuff-style headsets such as those used by construction workers.

- o Wear ear plugs, or plug up your ears with your fingers or cotton.

- o Develop the ability to shut out sound. This is not easy, but it is a learned ability. Go sit where other people are talking, perhaps in a waiting room, and experiment with ways not to hear them. For example, decide you will hear their words but their meaning will not penetrate your deeper mind. Or distract yourself with other thoughts.

For those women who prefer or require more noise in bathrooms, you can:

- o Turn up the volume on a CD or MP3 player, using headphones, of course.

- o Run a fan or air conditioner.

- o Use an MP3 player to record the noises in a busy restroom, like at a highway rest area or stadium, and then play it back in quiet restrooms – you could slowly decrease the volume over time to zero.

New inventions that may help

There are some devices already on the market that moderate sound in a bathroom stall and, perhaps, may represent the wave of the future.

Since the late 1970s, Japanese researchers have been on a mission to build a better toilet.

Many Japanese women are embarrassed at the thought that someone else can hear them while they are doing their business on the toilet. To cover the sound of bodily functions, some women repeatedly flushed public toilets while using them, wasting a large amount of water in the process.

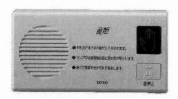

**Sound comes out
from this radio-like box**

Reprinted with permission of Toto Ltd.

In 1998, Toto Ltd., a leading Japanese toilet producer, introduced a product – the *"Sound Princess"* or *Otohime*™. After activation, it produces the sound of flushing water without the need for actual flushing. (See Appendix 2 for another photo and detailed description).

The creation of soundproof stalls

Soundproofing products are available to absorb and block noise. The addition of some kind of drywall material to walls and ceiling and the use of sound-absorbing liners and "soft materials," such as acoustic ceilings and padded carpet (rather than tile and laminates), are known to abate noise.

For further information, turn to Appendix 2 and read about "The Design of Women's Restrooms and Toilet Facilities".

Tips for Trips: Urinating While Traveling

The Issue

Paruretics find it difficult to urinate while traveling, when on moving vehicles (airplanes, trains, boats) and on motor trips.

Suggestions

o Learn to urinate on moving vehicles when bathrooms are least likely to be occupied.

o Take medication to help you retain urine longer.

o For road trips, consider taking along a portable toilet or learn to use an assistive device, such as a funnel, that can facilitate your ability to urinate outdoors.

Personal notes about traveling

One of my greatest passions in life is travel, and I consider myself fortunate to have visited many foreign countries on different continents. For me, the experience of being able to observe or "be in" other cultures has been both educational and enriching.

Despite having a rather severe case of paruresis, I made the conscious decision long ago to not let it prevent me from exploring the world. I gave myself a choice: I could either stay at home and urinate in peace, or I could refuse to be the victim of my disability and take some risks.

In the early days I managed to hold my urine for periods of up to 30 hours until I arrived at a bathroom in which I felt "safe." Once able to urinate, I was fine for the duration of the trip.

Later on, I discovered the alternative of self-catheterization, which provided a fallback position and gave me the freedom to more easily travel on long distance flights. Yet, as my anxiety grew and my emotional state deteriorated, even this knowledge was not enough to prevent me from constantly obsessing about restrooms prior to and during my trips. My fears about not being able to urinate led to self-fulfilling prophecies. Often it took me up to three days to be able to micturate on my own without having to use a catheter.

Travel became a bittersweet experience: a source of joy on one hand and an endurance test on the other.

Traveling with another person was especially problematic and became increasingly hard over the years. I needed my own private space, which eliminated staying at hostels and/or the bed-and-breakfast inns that offered only shared bathroom facilities.

When touring with a group of people by bus, I felt extra heavy time pressure. Restroom stops occur about every two to four hours – and all the women rush to use the bathroom at the same time, knowing they have to return to the bus within 10 to 15 minutes. Under those circumstances, I would not even attempt to go, instead choosing to hold my urine all day long until I returned to the sanctuary of my private room. After hearing reports of some arduous challenges I faced while on the road, several of my well-meaning friends began to question my rationale for traveling on "pleasure" trips. I did, too.

I can travel comfortably since my recovery from paruresis; so can you.

Suggestions

o Master the self-catheterization technique before you board any moving vehicle, or consider the use of an assistive device, such as wearing a urinary collection pouch or disposable urine bag. (See the section on "Other Assistive Devices" in Chapter 8.)

o Learn to urinate on moving vehicles when bathrooms are least likely to be occupied.

If, for example, you are traveling by airplane, the chances of your being able to urinate in a bathroom will most likely increase when other passengers are in their seats – when they're eating, watching a movie, or sleeping – and the aircraft is not experiencing turbulence. Plan your visits for these occasions.

o Count on taking a long time in the restroom. Carry a toiletry bag of items to keep you busy, such as a toothbrush or eye drops. If you think people are watching, make a point of showing you have your toiletries with you as you walk down the aisle.

o Take medication to help you retain urine for a longer period of time.

For long flights, consider the prudent use of Desmopressin Acetate, available in tablet or nasal spray form, which is prescribed to increase urine concentration and decrease urine production.

Normally, it is used to prevent nocturnal enuresis (bed wetting), but it has been found helpful for some paruretics.

o For road trips, consider taking along a portable toilet. The inexpensive ones – those with aluminum frame or constructed of durable corrugated paperboard – sell for about $15. Self-contained portable toilets of higher quality retail for about $70.

o If you can urinate while in a standing position or outdoors, try assistive devices, such as funnels or cones, to facilitate this process.

For further details, see Appendix 1, "Other Options When You Can't Urinate in a Restroom."

Foreign Travel

Not all bathrooms in foreign countries are created equal

Traveling in foreign countries can sometimes be daunting for those of us, non-paruretics and paruretics alike, who live in rich and highly-developed nations where we are used to invisible waste disposal systems. Sometimes we tend to forget that *the western-style flush toilet* with which we are so familiar is completely unknown in parts of the world that lack even running water, much less the ability to collect waste. Furthermore, contrary to our popular belief, not every country even believes that our type of toilet is such a terrific or sanitary idea!

In many parts of the world, the *squat (eastern-style) toilet* is more prevalent. It consists of an oblong hole, usually even with the floorboards, on either side of which are places to put your feet. They exist in every form: from rough, outhouse-style, standing-over-a-hole arrangements to tiled platforms with porcelain fixtures and a chain-pull flushing system.

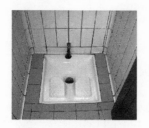

French squat toilet

Highly popular throughout most of Southeast Asia (China, Japan), the squat-style toilet is still somewhat common in public restrooms in southern and eastern Europe (including parts of France, Greece, Italy, and the Balkans) or when you venture off the beaten track.

In rural areas, particularly remote villages, people are likely to go into the fields to relieve themselves. Considered perfectly natural and normal by them, we paruretics would have to work hard at developing the ability to urinate alfresco.

Bathrooms have certain peculiarities in various countries. They are connected with national traditions and customs, climate conditions, and even inexplicable things. For example, in certain countries, you have to pay a fee before entering a toilet, whereas in other countries you are supposed to pay the fee after satisfying the call of nature. You may even have to pay for the toilet paper or bring your own. Many public toilets in Europe are automatic: you can go in if you put a coin in the slot and you can go out only if you flush. In certain bathrooms you may see the list of prices converted in all currencies of the world.

The bathroom experience can vary even within the same country, ranging from the very modern to very primitive. In the western parts of Turkey, such as in Istanbul, visitors find mostly western facilities. However, the further east you travel into Turkey's interior, the more squat toilets become the norm. In Korea, hotels and some other public areas have western toilets. However, usually only squat toilets are available at bus stops – sometimes they are unisex, with urinals and women's stalls in the same enclosed room.

Here are some general rules of thumb:

o Modern facilities generally contain the best restrooms. Look for them in fancy hotel lobbies, large restaurants, cafes and bars, department and retail chain stores, college campuses, shopping malls, and popular tourist attractions.

o Good facilities are likely to be found in major city centers that have museums, art galleries and civic buildings.

o The chance of finding adequate bathroom facilities in public areas such as schools, train stations, airports, etc. is probably better than average but still iffy.

o Most, but not all of, McDonalds and Starbucks have toilets that are clean, well-maintained and free.

o In general, bathrooms in developed European countries are a delight. They contain private cubicles with ceiling-to-floor walls and doors, no cracks around the doors, and good locks.

o Bathrooms in Japan (and some other Asian countries) are unique because squat-style toilets may coexist with often futuristic "western-style" ones.

The Japanese tend to pay attention to bathroom etiquette and are known for their clean toilets and outstanding standards of hygiene.

But, still, lines can be found waiting to use bathrooms.

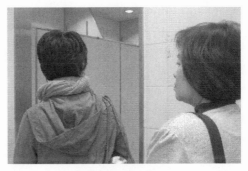

Public park in Tokyo

Photo by Carol Olmert

Research bathrooms in foreign countries before visiting

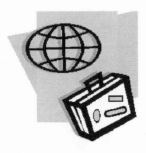

Before taking a trip to a foreign country, it is useful to learn as much as possible about restroom facilities there.

As long as you know what to watch out for and how to prepare yourself, you can probably successfully manage the most difficult of bathroom situations.

Several Internet sites provide detailed information on restrooms in specific countries. Some allow you to trade observations and frustrations about your restroom experiences with others.

Excellent descriptions of bathrooms in other countries can be found at *The Bathroom Diaries*™, www.thebathroomdiaries.com, which rates 9,000-plus public bathrooms in more than 100 countries and provides a wealth of information to both travelers and urban dwellers. Equally valuable are several other websites:

www.americanrestroom.org/pr/support/reports.htm

www.biz2web.com/grant/Bathrooms.htm

www.cromwell-intl.com/toilet/

www.darkcreek.com/toilets

www.icbe.org/pages/international.shtml
(bathroom etiquette around the world)

www.mizpee.com

www.publictoilets.org/pt

www.restroomratings.com

www.ricksteves.com/graffiti/archives/toilets.htm (Europe only)

www.theplumber.com/russiantoilets.html (Russia)

www.travelblog.org/Forum/Threads/2356-1.html

www.urinal.net

www.virtualtourist.com

www.worldtoilet.info

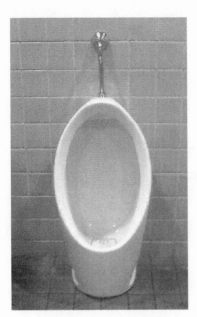

**Little boy's urinal
in female restroom, Japan**

Photo by Carol Olmert

Information about toilets in Japan is also widespread. New toilet technology is constantly being introduced and includes heated seats, a spray for cleaning oneself (with adjustments for regulating water temperature), and water pressure adjustment jets – all contain an array of instructions (always in Japanese, but sometimes illustrated with pictures). Many women's restrooms even include a small urinal for use by young boys. Good descriptions of these features can be found at www.answers.com/topic/japanese-toilet and www.japan-guide.com/e/e2003.html

Chapter Eight
Survival Skills: Ways to Empty Your Bladder

As indicated in Chapter 7, we paruretics have a number of "work-arounds" at our disposal. Again, remember that they address the symptom only, not the problem.

By strict definition, survival skills involve *anything* you can do to be able to urinate, including distraction, doing mental arithmetic, masking sounds with headphones, finding "safe" bathrooms, etc. Recovery skills, on the other hand, promote desensitization and increased functioning over the long term.

Catheterization – Finding Immediate Relief

A survival tool

Catheterization refers to the process of inserting a slim tube (a catheter) into the opening of your urinary tract for purposes of releasing urine. It can either be performed by a health care practitioner, someone who has been trained in its use, or by yourself, assuming you receive proper instruction.

Self-catheterization can be considered the ultimate escape route, the surefire way to find immediate relief when urination is otherwise impossible. Once taught and comfortable with the process (this may require some practice), you will have the assurance that you can urinate anywhere. Sometimes, the mere fact of having this mental safety net may be liberating enough to let you overcome anticipatory anxiety and begin recovery work.

Catheterization supplies typically consist of:

o   A sterile catheter, which comes in various sizes and materials.

o   A water-soluble lubricant, such as K-Y Jelly™, Surgilube™, or Lubrifax™ , which you apply to the tip of the catheter prior to inserting it. (Do **not** use Vaseline or petroleum jelly because they can plug the catheter.)

o   An antibacterial wipe or disinfectant, which normally comes in individual packets and is used to cleanse the vaginal area prior to inserting the catheter.

o   Soapy wash cloth and clean dry towel.

o   A plastic tray (or an actual toilet bowl) into which the released urine will flow.

o   A hand mirror if required.

o   A catheter storage kit, e.g., a small plastic bag with Ziploc® or tie closure or even a toothbrush holder.

CISC for short-term relief

Clean Intermittent Self Catheterization (CISC) refers to the technique that is used only for the short term, as opposed to the in-dwelling type that is retained for longer periods of time. First adopted in 1970 as a home self-technique, it is performed regularly by thousands of people worldwide to manage bladder function, especially among those with neurological disorders, and may be necessary for women after certain gynecological and other surgeries or following childbirth. Some women use catheterization to manage urinary incontinence.

The goal of intermittent catheterization is to prevent urinary tract infections while still completely emptying the bladder. The procedure must be sterile, and the catheter must be free from bacteria. You can reduce the risk for a Urinary Tract Infection (UTI) by using antiseptic techniques for insertion and catheter care.

CISC catheters are straight tubes and more rigid than in-dwelling catheters, making insertion a little easier. They may be a clear plastic or a softer red rubber material. After urine drainage, the catheter is removed from the body, cleaned, and stored.

Remember, all catheters are *not* created equal. They vary in tip shape and the size of the tube, which is measured according to the French (Fr) scale (about one-third of a millimeter). The usual size of the outside circumference is 14 Fr, 16 Fr, or 18 Fr, but generally is smaller for women. For example, if you're of petite stature, you may require one whose outside diameter is less, e.g., I use a 10 Fr, which is considered an adolescent size.

If you decide to try a catheter, you will need to experiment to find which kind and design works best for you, as well as understand its strengths and limitations. Further discussion on catheterization can be found on the IPA's website at http://www.paruresis.org/catheter.htm.

Most insurance plans will not cover the cost of catheters, but they can be purchased at a nominal cost and without a prescription from medical supply companies, often on the Internet. Some allow you to sample a few kinds and/or sizes, such as www.cathforfree.com, and others will allow you to purchase catheters in small quantities.

How to catheterize yourself

To perform Clean Intermittent Self Catheterization (CISC), you must learn the basic location of the important urological landmarks.

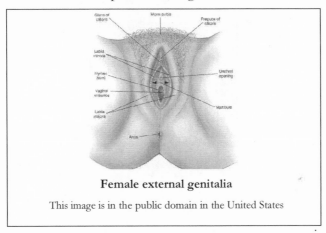

Female external genitalia

This image is in the public domain in the United States

It is highly recommended that you be taught by a knowledgeable health care practitioner, preferably a female, before attempting the process by yourself.

For those women who need further instruction in urinary self-catheterization, a self-instruction video is now available. Entitled *Guide to Self-Catheterization for Women,* it is available through the Rehabilitation Institute of Chicago at http://lifecenter.ric.org/content/3509/index.html?topic=1&subtopic=273.

The following section contains general information about self-catheterization for women, adapted from various websites and augmented by my personal notes.

How to perform Clean Intermittent Self-Catheterization(CISC)

1. Get into a position that is most comfortable for you. Choose beforehand if you want to release your urine into a catheter tray or a toilet bowl. That decision will influence the length (shorter or longer) of the catheter you buy.

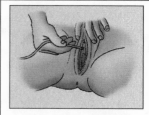

Insertion of a urinary catheter in a female

Used by permission of John Samellas.
© 2007 MedSelfEd, Inc.

   Author's note: As a matter of preference and/or convenience, some women may perform CISC standing beside the toilet with one foot resting on its rim. Others find it easier to do so while lying in a supine (on the back) position, emptying urine into a catheter tray. For practicality, I recommend that you learn the method by sitting on a toilet, maybe backwards for starters, to ensure greater access to the urethral opening (meatus). This position makes it easier to identify the urethral opening by feel and allows you to empty your urine directly into a toilet bowl. You will need a shorter catheter to accomplish this.

2. Gather all your equipment and supplies, placing them on a clean surface within easy reach. Arrange clothing so it is out of the way.

3. Wash your hands with soap and water, and dry them thoroughly before you begin. It's one of the most important steps in self-catheterization. Clean the entire vaginal area with the throw-away antibacterial wipes or disinfectant.

   Author's note: Wipe from front to back to prevent contaminating the area with fecal contents.

4. Lubricate the catheter.

   Author's note: Apply water-soluble lubricant, such as K-Y Jelly™ or Lubrifax™, to the insertion end of the catheter. Lubricate about three inches at the tip of the tubing. Self-lubricating catheters can also be purchased (for further information consult http://www.astratechusa.com).

5. Locate the urethral opening (meatus). It can be found below the clitoris and above the vagina (see diagram). To do so, spread your thighs apart and use your non-dominant hand (i.e., left hand for right-handed women). Separate your vaginal lips (labia) with the second and fourth finger, while using the middle finger to reveal or feel for the opening.

Author's note: A device is now available that makes it much easier to locate the meatus. Called *The Asta Cath*® Female Catheter Guide, it contains three alignment holes that provide proper alignment for a 14 Fr or smaller catheter to pass into the bladder for emptying. It cleans easily with soap and water, is dishwasher-safe, and latex-free. For further information, consult medical supply companies, such as Bruce Medical Supply at http://www.brucemedical.com/ab10001.html.

If you have difficulty finding the urethral opening at first, using a small hand mirror may help – but don't become dependent on it since it will limit your flexibility. Such mirrors are available from medical supply companies, such as Sammons Preston at http://www.sammonspreston.com/Supply/Product.asp?Leaf_Id=6225.

6. Hold the catheter in your dominant hand and, slowly and gently, insert it into the urethral opening, guiding it upward. Do not rush the procedure.

   Author's note: If you have difficulty placing the catheter and become nervous, stop, take a deep breath, and then start over. It is not uncommon to have difficulty the first few times. If you feel pain or resistance with the passage of a catheter, you may not have used enough lubrication. Do not force the catheter at any time. If you accidentally insert the catheter into the vagina (easy to do), remove it and wash it with soap and water or use a clean catheter.

7. Once the catheter has been inserted about two to three inches (eight centimeters) past the opening, urine will begin to flow. Breathe slowly and relax your muscles.

8. Once the urine flow starts, continue to advance the catheter another one inch (three centimeters) and hold it in place until the urine flow stops and the bladder is empty.

9. Withdraw the catheter in small steps, gently and slowly, to make sure the entire bladder empties. Using toilet paper, wipe from front to back only.

10. Readjust your clothing.

11. If the catheter is disposable and single-use, discard it right away. If it is reusable, wash the catheter completely with soap and water for 10 seconds and rinse well. Place it on a clean cloth to air dry. When dry, store the catheter in a clean and dry container, such as a make-up bag or a Ziploc® bag until the next time it is used.

    Author's note: I store mine in a special compartment of my purse or fanny pack.

A CISC catheter may be reused for two to four weeks. It may be helpful to soak the catheter in a white vinegar solution once a week to control odor and remove thick mucus deposits. Other cleaning or sterilization techniques may be recommended by your health care provider if infection occurs frequently.

A cautionary note

You may experience a slight burning sensation or discomfort after you urinate for the first few times following self-catheterization. Do not be alarmed! Urethritis (inflammation of the urethra) may result from using catheters that are too large, inserted with insufficient lubrication, or inserted improperly. Some female paruretics claim the use of Advil™ prior to self-catheterization can reduce the possibility of discomfort.

Warning: If you continue to notice any of the following symptoms, contact your doctor as soon as possible.

o Sudden urge to urinate (doctors call this "urgency").

o Blood on the catheter.

o Need to urinate more frequently.

o Pain, burning, or cramps during or immediately after urination ("dysuria").

o Feeling that the bladder will not empty completely.

o Urge to urinate during sleeping hours ("nocturia").

o Cloudy or foul-smelling urine, which may indicate the presence of pus ("pyuria").

o Blood in the urine ("hematuria").

o Bladder discomfort during sexual intercourse.

o Lower abdominal cramps, soreness, or pain.

o Backache.

o Fever.

o Loss of bladder control ("urinary incontinence") may be a symptom in older women.

You may have developed a Urinary Tract Infection (UTI) or possibly injured your urethra or bladder.

What if a Urinary Tract Infection (UTI) Develops?

Women are significantly more likely to experience urinary tract infections (UTIs or cystitis) than men. Nearly one in three women will have had at least one UTI episode requiring antimicrobial therapy by the age of 24 years. Almost half of all women will experience one UTI during their lifetime (Foxman, 2002).

Cystitis is uncomfortable but usually responds well to treatment. A mild case may resolve on its own without treatment. In order to reduce the associated burning and urgency, a medication called Phenazopyridine hydrochloride (commonly called Uristat™) is available without prescription at your local pharmacy. One side effect may be discoloration of urine, which turns from yellow to reddish-orange. In addition, acidifying medications, such as ascorbic acid, may be recommended to decrease the concentration of bacteria in the urine.

Antibacterial drugs can be prescribed by your personal physician to alleviate the symptoms of UTIs.

Author's note: I use antibacterials as a preventative measure, though this practice is controversial and should be discussed with your physician first. Prophylactic use of antibacterial agents may lead to the development of drug-resistant bacteria.

The choice of drug and length of treatment depend on the patient's history and the urine tests that identify the offending bacteria. The sensitivity test is especially useful in helping the doctor select the most effective drug. It is important that you finish the entire course of prescribed antibiotics.

According to the National Kidney and Urologic Diseases Information Clearinghouse (NKUDIC) ("National Kidney and Urologic Diseases Information Clearinghouse", n.d.), the drugs most often used to treat routine, uncomplicated UTIs are:

o Trimethoprim/sulfamethoxazole (Bactrim™, Septra™, Cotrim™). Patients who are allergic to these sulfonamides may be treated with drugs within the trimethoprim class (Trimpex™, Primsole™, Proloprim™) alone.

o Amoxicillin (Amoxil™, Trimox™, Wymox™).

o Nitrofurantoin (Macrodantin™, Furadantin™).

o Ampicillin (Omnipen™, Polycillin™, Principen™, Totacillin™).

o A class of drugs called quinolones includes four drugs approved in recent years for treating UTIs. These drugs include ofloxacin (Floxin™), norfloxacin (Noroxin™), ciprofloxacin (Cipro™), and trovafloxin (Trovan™).

Comments from other female paruretics about self-catheterization

Better than a full bladder

It does not hurt, just mildly uncomfortable but not as bad as having a full bladder. Be sure to use the K-Y™ lubricant. I ran out last time and irritated my urethra when I inserted it with just water as a lubricant. My urethra burned for a day or two after that. It just takes practice.

Some helpful suggestions

I do self-cath in an emergency but experience some discomfort and burning, so I really try to save it for the times when I see no other way out. It has been a life-saver just to have it, though. I also highly recommend lubrication, and one other thing: it is quite awkward to SEE the opening to the urethra, and I have had more success when I FEEL it with my finger and then put the cath in rather than trying to bend my body in a strange position and then put it in.

Life changed in five minutes

About four years ago a gynecologist taught me to self-cath. He cured me!!!! In five minutes....my life changed forever. I have had no UTIs in four years...and no pain whatsoever...so for me, personally, I recommend the cath. My life is wonderful now.

Other Assistive Devices

Besides self-catheterization, some women find other non-invasive urinary products that may be of some help in bladder emptying. The list includes:

o Urinary collection bags.

o Disposable urinal bags.

o Funnels (as an aid if you learn to urinate while standing up).

o Portable urinals.

o Portable toilets and privacy tents.

One product, a urinary pouch, provides an alternative to restroom use. When attached to your inner thigh, it is completely hidden beneath loose fitting jeans or pants. A valve at the bottom of the pouch can be opened to empty urine into a toilet bowl.

Disposable and portable urinal bags are also sold. They contain absorbent material that solidifies the urine in 5 to 10 seconds, making it convenient and safe to keep (leakproof, puncture resistant, and odorless) until there is an opportunity for disposal.

Other products have been found to be especially beneficial to women who travel or find themselves in outdoor situations. They are generally referred to as female urination devices or female urination aids, such as a funnel or medical-grade tubing which can enable females to urinate through the fly of their clothes while standing. For further instructions about how to urinate while standing up, access http://ganimede_x.tripod.com/stp.html.

A few female portable urinals have recently been introduced that can be used while lying flat on your back, seated or standing. They are designed to carry easily and make good travel companions in a car, boat, or when camping.

Portable toilets and privacy tents may provide an alternative for those who seek peace and quiet when they want to urinate, especially in outdoor situations. Some people deliberately purchase some sort of van in which they can close off a private area for a "porta potty."

All these alternatives are examined in greater detail in Appendix 1, "Other Options When You Can't Urinate in a Restroom."

There is a time and place when crutches are useful, even necessary. However, at some point, in order to heal completely, you need to throw them away and begin a treatment program.

The most effective way of treating paruresis to date has been the use of Cognitive-Behavioral Therapy (CBT). For some, this method of treatment has been enhanced by the use of Medications and/or Breathing, Breath Holding, and Relaxation Techniques as part of a comprehensive approach.

This next section will explain each of these tools in depth.

Cognitive-Behavioral Therapy (CBT)

Cognitive-Behavioral Therapy (CBT) has two main components:

o   Cognitive Restructuring: To change your distorted thinking.

o   Behavioral: To learn and practice graduated exposure techniques (systematic desensitization).

Cognitive Restructuring is a term used to describe a way of identifying and replacing fear-promoting, irrational beliefs with more realistic and functional ones. The basic premise is that faulty assumptions contribute to your anxiety; these thoughts must be identified and restructured. Cognitive therapy is not merely positive thinking but is the pursuit of accurate and realistic thinking (Robbins, April 10, 2007).

The behavioral component is based on systematic desensitization, also called **Graduated Exposure.** The concept involves gradually and repetitively attempting to urinate in the presence of others, in closer and closer proximity and in situations ranging from those which feel "safe" to more challenging ones. In other words, you learn to face, rather than avoid, your fears. Over a period of time, your brain is re-wired to realize that urinating when others are nearby is not threatening or dangerous.

CBT requires strong dedication and patience on the part of the paruretic. It is possible to learn and practice graduated exposure exercises independently or with a friend. However, if you're the type of person who finds it hard to start and keep at something, you may benefit from the assistance of a group or a trained therapist.

Finding professional help

One person who has been of great help to female paruretics and who also serves on the IPA's Board of Advisors is:

Ruth Lippin, LMSW
782 West End Avenue #42
New York NY 10025
212.666.1062
ruthlippin@aol.com

To find a certified cognitive therapist in your area, consult the Academy of Cognitive Therapy at www.academyofct.org/Library/CertifiedMembers/Index.asp?FolderID=1 137&SessionID={C8392E59-B4E4-4C9E-BC11-01F908EE3D41}&RLMsg=&SP= or the Anxiety Disorders Association of America at http://community.adaa.org/eweb/DynamicPage.aspx?Site=adaa&WebKe y=ce66a0ec-3e19-437d-836b-f180fcdf6814.

In order to recover from paruresis, you need to be fully committed to the practice of these graduated exposure exercises. You need to acquire the discipline to schedule practice sessions on a regular basis – not because you just happen to be at a shopping mall or department store where a bathroom is conveniently located. The importance of regular practice cannot be emphasized enough.

Cognitive restructuring: The basic premise

o Recognize the connection between thoughts and feelings.

o We chatter to ourselves constantly.

o Identify thoughts and attitudes that are distorted, exaggerated or illogical.

o Challenge these automatic thoughts.

o Substitute more realistic and positive thoughts and beliefs, which will reduce painful feelings.

o Prepare for relapse: we are constantly in a state of growth, and new challenges may cause us to revert to previously learned behavior(s).

Throughout this book, I have included some examples of Cognitive Restructuring techniques under the headings of *"Challenge Your Thinking"*. In the following section, I will provide you with a more detailed explanation.

People who are able to effectively benefit from this technique are able to regard their beliefs somewhat dispassionately, to stand away from them and look at the basis for holding them in the first place.

Example: If you feel like "someone is going to judge me," realize this is a thought, not a feeling. A thought is a hypothesis that can be tested with evidence. It is a conclusion you drew that you need to challenge to see if it is accurate.

Dr. John Cook, a psychologist who practices cognitive therapy and the founder of Aegis Psychological Services, Inc. in Victoria, British Columbia, describes the four steps that need to be completed in cognitive restructuring. The following excerpt is reprinted with his permission (Cook, 2006).

Step One

Elicit automatic thoughts

Automatic thoughts are habitual ways of thinking and generally occur spontaneously. You can use some of the following techniques to help elicit them.

A. Focus on an image, such as a toilet seat, and ask for whatever words come to mind.

B. Use your imagination to mentally recreate a situation you face in a bathroom. Ask yourself what thoughts come to mind or what you think others might be thinking when you approach a bathroom.

C. The next time you approach a public restroom, notice and write down your thoughts.

Step Two

Identify underlying irrational beliefs

Examine the automatic thoughts for any cognitive distortions (*"self-talk"*) you may find and look for common themes. Keep a detailed diary to record your thoughts, feelings, and actions when problem situations around bathrooms arise. This journal will help to make you aware of your maladaptive thoughts and to show their consequences on your behavior.

Irrational beliefs that underlie automatic thoughts are all based on flawed or faulty logic.

Here are some examples:

A. <u>Emotional reasoning</u> is mood-state dependent thinking based on the assumption that feeling something strongly necessarily makes it true, e.g., "If I am nervous, then I must be performing terribly."

B. <u>Over generalization</u> is the use of a single negative event as evidence for a never-ending pattern of negative events, e.g., "Michael said he didn't have time for coffee with me yesterday … I'll never get a date with him."

C. <u>All-or-nothing (black & white) thinking</u> is seen in statements that use absolute terms such as *always, never, completely, totally or perfectly* to suggest you are a failure if your performance falls short of these standards, e.g., "I am a failure unless I can always urinate in a stall with a woman sitting in an adjacent one."

D. <u>Should statements</u> are statements that suggest a desire to change some reality when the only real choice is between accepting or not accepting it, e.g., "My manager should show greater appreciation for the hard work I do."

E. <u>Jumping to conclusions</u> happens when negative interpretations are made of events without sufficient supporting evidence.

F. <u>Fortune telling</u> occurs as unfounded, usually dire predictions that are made as if they are already fact, e.g., a mildly paruretic woman, unable to urinate in a public restroom during a concert, says "I probably won't be able to urinate at tomorrow evening's performance, either."

G. <u>Mind-reading</u> is a prediction about other people's thoughts or behaviors that is made without checking them out. It sometimes represents the projection of one person's thoughts/feelings onto another person, e.g., "She must think I'm weird because I spend so much time in the restroom."

H. <u>Selective negative focus</u> is focusing on the negative aspect of a situation while ignoring the positive, e.g., a student who fails the oral part of an exam but passes the written with an 'A' says, "I really messed up that exam."

I. <u>Disqualifying the positive</u> is a rejection of positive experiences by insisting they "don't count," e.g., a student who fails the oral part of an exam but passes the written with an 'A' says, "I usually do well on written exams, that's not what is important to me."

J. <u>Magnification and minimization</u> are also referred to as the "binocular trick" because it happens when we enlarge our shortcomings or someone else's accomplishments while shrinking our accomplishments or someone else's shortcomings, e.g., "I'm not half the woman my sister is. Everything she touches seems to turn to gold."

K. <u>Catastrophizing</u> is a building up of consequences to an event so that they seem insufferable or particularly horrible, e.g., "If I don't urinate right now, I'll have to stay home and cancel my date with David. If this continues, I'm going to end up a lonely old maid."

L. <u>Personalization</u> happens when we interpret an event or a situation as having special meaning (usually negative) for only ourselves, e.g., "If I hadn't hired on with this company, they never would have gone bankrupt."

Step Three

Challenge the irrational beliefs

Questions to ask when experiencing stressful automatic thoughts:

o Am I jumping to conclusions?

o Evaluate the thought: what is the evidence for it and against it?

o   Am I exaggerating or overemphasizing a negative aspect of the situation?

o   Am I "catastrophizing"?

o   How do I know it will happen?

o   So what if it happens?

o   Is it really as bad as it seems?

o   Is it to my advantage to maintain this appraisal?

o   Is there another way to look at the situation?

Once you have identified the irrational beliefs, begin to refute them by examining the evidence for the thought and by looking for alternative explanations.

Questions can be used to refute irrational beliefs in two ways:

1.   Those dealing with how certain we are a particular outcome will occur are referred to as probability dispute handles.

2.   Those that concern the worst thing that could happen and how bad that is are called coping dispute handles.

Here are some examples of each:

Probability Dispute Handles	**Coping Dispute Handles**
o What are the other possible outcomes?	o What is the evidence to suggest the consequences will be disastrous?
o What evidence do we have that _____ will happen?	o Could there be any other explanation?
o Does _____ have to equal or lead to _____?	o Is _____ really so important that my whole future depends on it?
o What has happened in the past? Any exceptions?	o Does _____'s opinion reflect that of everyone else?
o What are the chances of it happening/happening again?	

Step Four

Replace the irrational beliefs with suitable alternatives

Often the replacements for automatic thoughts become evident in the course of refuting the irrational beliefs on which they are based. Your challenge now is to devise rational alternative thoughts based on the information you have acquired.

o   Replace irrational beliefs with truthful, rational statements.

o   Write down a more positive coping thought that is more consistent with the facts and evidence.

An example of one female paruretic's process

First, she analyzed her thoughts:

I think they are going to hear me and if the flow is weak they will compare and wonder what my problem is. They are going to wonder why I'm taking so long and why I'm not peeing yet. Someone is going to see me through the cracks. The person next to me feels too close for me to relax. Uh oh, what if I can't go? I feel like an oddball. Everyone else pees with no problem; so why can't I? I have a flawed conscience, and God might not let these muscles relax till I get things right.

*Then she counteracted her distorted thinking and
reminded herself of some basic truths:*

So what if they hear me? So what if they wonder? They are thinking about their own stuff, not concentrating on me. It's easier to see out of the cracks than into them. They are only checking to see if anyone is in there, they don't care who it is. I have the right to take as long as I want, and the right to be comfortable. Everyone has their problems; this is not the end of the world. I can catheterize myself if I need to. I've peed with an unresolved conscience before, and there have been times I couldn't pee with a resolved conscience – hello? And within the past year: hmmm. Maybe I CAN. I can at least try. I'm going to tell whoever I'm with I might be a while because I have trouble. My walkman might help. I can have more than one chance. I'm not alone with this problem. I'm generally not an oddball, but if this is the only oddity, well okay, then.

The behavioral component: The basic premise

The behavioral component is based on **systematic desensitization**, also called **graduated exposure therapy.** Here you create a hierarchy of feared situations and start to allow yourself to experience them. You begin with low-level anxiety situations and then gradually move up your hierarchy.

This must be done *in reality*, not just as visualization. Each session of exposure therapy involves several attempts at briefly urinating.

Before you begin, read the following caveats:

o "Fluid loading" is a key step in graduated exposure therapy, and because it is contrary to the normal pattern that paruretics have of controlling their liquid intake, it might be scary for some. Prior to each practice session, an individual is encouraged to drink enough water so that she can urinate as many times as possible during the session. It is important to note that you should drink only enough liquid to reach a moderate state of urgency to urinate.

o I strongly recommend taking an IPA Weekend Workshop or Intensive Workshop because I believe you really have to see and experience the graduated exposure process in practice before you can apply it. Additionally you will benefit from the opportunity to share your experience of paruresis with others, as well as gain new insights.

> **Author's note**: To learn exactly what happens at an IPA Workshop, read the section on "Take an IPA Workshop" in Chapter 10. The schedule of IPA workshops appears on the organization's website at http://www.shybladder.org/workshops.php.

o It is helpful to have a safe backup plan in mind. On very rare occasions, people with shy bladder find themselves unable to initiate urination during their practice session and then are unable to urinate when they return home. Knowing how to self-catheterize can be of great benefit. If you find yourself "locking up," seek medical attention immediately to gain relief.

o It is best to avoid the deliberate use of background noise, such as running a water faucet or blower or having a television set on, when practicing in a bathroom since much of the exposure treatment will likely have to be repeated once the background noise is eliminated.

o At the end of each practice session, reward yourself. Give yourself something – a foot massage, a walk, or a treat.

Step One

Find a partner to work with

This person can be a trained behavioral therapist, someone from an IPA support group or workshop, a buddy, a close friend, or family member. The person does not have to be a paruretic, as long as s/he is non-judgmental and offers you comfort.

Note: If you do not have a partner, practice urinating in restrooms that are empty at first, then move on to situations where one person is present. Then progress to a slightly more crowded restroom. Once you are consistently successful with a few people present in the restroom, advance to more crowded restrooms. Useful restrooms for this practice include those at interstate rest areas, busy airports, sporting events, concerts, or theaters. See below for an example of how to practice by yourself.

Step Two

Construct hierarchy scales

Take out a fresh piece of paper and begin to write down your personal hierarchy, one which will be unique to you. Using a 0-10 scale, come up with those scenarios in which you have an easy time using the bathroom (for example, Level 0 might be at home alone) and those in which you have a difficult time urinating (for example, Level 10 might be using a crowded public restroom at a concert during intermission). The bottom of your hierarchy will be the baseline, a situation in which you could reasonably expect to be able to go; the top of the hierarchy will be what you most want to achieve.

Create a similar behavioral hierarchy for your desensitization practices, unique to you. Level 0 might mean going into a bathroom and coming back out. Level 1 could be going into the bathroom and washing your hands. Level 10 might be sitting in a stall with a line of impatient women knocking on the door demanding immediate entrance.

Remember, this list must be tailored specifically to your feared situations and consists of small incremental steps.

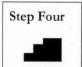

Step Three

Begin fluid loading

In order to use exposure therapy, a substantial amount of urine is needed. Drink plenty of fluids (water is best) prior to the start of a practice session. Usually drinking about one quart of water one hour before the practice session is optimal, but, of course, that depends on body size. Some people may require more water or more time to pass before they feel the strong need to urinate. Most people with shy bladder are more successful if their need to urinate is high at the time of the practice session. Occasionally, some people have more trouble when they are very urgent, so experimentation may be necessary.

Some find it helpful to use a scale to record how strongly they feel the need to urinate. Again, a 0-10 point scale works well, starting with Level 0 indicating no urgency and rising to Level 10, which equals extreme urgency. It will probably work out best to start practice sessions only after you rate your urgency at Level 7 or above.

Step Four

Begin a practice session

For many people, it is helpful to start the initial practice session in an isolated private restroom. Practice can begin by having your partner stand at enough of a distance from you where you think you will be able to urinate.

- o For some, that might mean outside of the restroom with the door closed.

- o For others, that could mean standing at the end of a long corridor, if, for example, you start your practice in a hotel room or office setting.

- o For others, that could mean having your partner stand outside of the building.

Remember: you are in control of your own experience, so you tell your partner *exactly* where to position her/himself. This is not a contest, so make sure you start where you are comfortable. Once you and your partner are in place, you should attempt to urinate.

Use the following two "rules" to guide you:

○ The ***three-second*** and the ***three-minute rules***: If you are able to void, allow urine to flow for approximately three seconds so that you have enough left for the next practice during this same session. That may be hard to do, especially for older women whose bladder muscles may have loosened.

After successfully completing the urination trial, meet up with your partner and take a short break of approximately three minutes, after which you should repeat that trial for a second time. If your partner is also a paruretic who wants to practice, switch roles after that second successful trial.

○ The ***two-minute rule***: If you have trouble initiating urination, wait at the toilet for two minutes before giving up and taking a break. If you feel that you are just about to urinate after two minutes, wait up to two minutes more before walking away.

Usually waiting beyond four minutes is not helpful. If you cannot urinate, take a short three-minute break before trying again. Have your partner move back to where you last urinated, and then once you can void again (twice), move slowly toward the point where you last weren't able to go.

Step Five

Have your partner move incrementally closer to you

Once you can start your urine stream, have your partner slowly (that could mean an inch or a foot at a time, you decide) move closer to you as you climb the hierarchy of feared situations that you established. You can also give specific directions to your partner about what you want her/him to do during a practice session, e.g., "I want you to sit two feet away from me and read a book." Make sure you repeat each session twice.

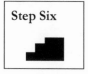

Step Six

Follow four general guidelines

1. **Decide how often to practice**: It is best to practice often, preferably several times per week. For some women, this may seem like an impossible assignment. However, in order to climb your hierarchy, you must treat your recovery as if it were a job. The real answer to the question, *"how much should I practice?"* is *"how soon do you*

want to recover?" Longer sessions are generally more helpful than shorter sessions. About one hour is best, with the goal of getting several practice trials in each of these one-hour sessions.

You may also need to continually fluid load during your session to have enough pressure and urine to continue practicing the entire time.

2. **Understand that your experiences may vary from one practice session to another.** If you have trouble initiating one day and then no problem the next, do not be overly concerned; many people experience inconsistency in their progress. It's normal and nothing to worry about.

3. **Do not use words like "success" or "failure" to describe your practice session.** Acknowledge yourself for having the courage to try. Your "success" is that you practiced, not that you were able to urinate.

4. **Find the halfway point.** If you do have trouble with a given step in the exposure process, try and find the halfway point between what worked previously and where you are having difficulty. One of the most frequent mistakes people make in doing graduated exposure work is to move too quickly up their behavioral hierarchy. In fact, *just a few inches can make the difference*, since our boundaries between unsafe and safe situations are so clearly delineated in our own minds.

The number of sessions required. You should expect the self-treatment to require at least eight and perhaps as many as 12 sessions, or the duration of a weekend workshop, before you notice significant improvement. Of course, you could require fewer or more than this range specifies. It is important to know that this treatment has been helpful to many people, but there is no guarantee that it will help you. Data from the IPA indicate that about 80 to 90% of paruretics using these techniques are helped to a significant degree. Finally, if your self-treatment fails, consult a trained behavioral therapist for help.

Putting it all together – A hierarchy for practice

The hierarchy will look different for each person – what is a small step for one may be a big step for another. Let's say your ultimate goal is to be able to urinate in a small (2-3 stalls) bathroom with a friend sitting next to you chatting and you having a strong need to go. You prefer solo practice or lack a practice partner. Here's what your hierarchy might look like:

0. The bathroom in your home or apartment, no one present, medium urgency.

1. The handicapped stall in a large public restroom with no one present, low urgency, and your home a 10 minute drive away if needed.

2. A large public restroom with no one present and lots of noise (if you prefer quiet bathrooms) or little noise (if you prefer noisy bathrooms), medium urgency.

3. A large public restroom in which there are two or three other women present, but they're sitting far away from you, medium urgency (bring them closer to you the next time).

4. A large public restroom in which there are two or three other women present, but one is in an adjacent stall, low urgency.

5. A medium-sized public restroom (5-6 cubicles) with no one present, high urgency.

6. A medium-sized public restroom (5-6 cubicles) with someone sitting two stalls apart, medium urgency.

7. A medium-sized public restroom (5-6 cubicles) with someone sitting next to you, low urgency.

8. A small public restroom (2-3 stalls) with no one present, low urgency.

9. A small public restroom (2-3 stalls) with a friend; you sit in one cubicle and she in the other, begin conversation, medium urgency.

10. A small public restroom (2-3 stalls) with a friend; you sit in one cubicle and she in the other, begin conversation, high urgency.

Other ways to practice exposure

Long-term improvement is totally dependent on the practice of the form of graduated exposure described above. This protocol is oriented toward learning to urinate around others.

However, another application recommended by IPA co-founder Carl Robbins can be equally important. Promoting desensitization, it involves embracing your fears without resistance. It entails doing the opposite to get rid of what you don't want or fear and taking it to the extreme. Here, the goal is not to eliminate your hesitancy; rather it's to face your fear of hesitancy. In these exposures, you put aside any hope or attainment of success when urinating around others.

According to Robbins, the fear that paruretics have is not the fear of going; rather the core fear is about not going and other people noticing it. The fear of NOT going makes you try harder to go, which, in turn, makes it more difficult to go. Studies have shown that the act of "trying" or "trying too hard" or "obsessing" can produce stress or anxiety. So, when it's okay to fail, you will be more likely to succeed (Robbins, November 11, 2006).

The exposure exercises that Robbins recommends require you to actually confront your fears through prolonged and intentional exposure to them. You deliberately and consciously invite your anxiety – you allow it to rise, peak and subside while exposing yourself to public non-urination – and simply wait for it to go away on its own. You become an "impartial observer" of your thoughts and emotions. By not resisting your restroom anxiety and developing a fundamentally new relationship with it, you learn to embrace and accept your fears.

These exercises are based on the psychological concepts of "Paradoxical Intention" (developed by logotherapist Victor Frankl) and "The Ironic Process" (a term coined by psychologist Daniel M. Wegner). Ascher applied these techniques to treat male paruretics in a 1979 study (Wells & Giannetti, p.160). They are consistent with the practice of mindfulness and a new approach to fighting anxiety (Acceptance and Commitment Therapy, or ACT), as well as the long-standing principles of habituation and desensitization.

The following three exercises are designed to be performed while you're in a public restroom.

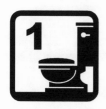 *Three minutes in a cubicle.* Walk into a stall without any intention of urinating. Do this when you do not need to urinate or with a low level of urgency. Take your mind into the restroom as well – but do not give your thoughts much attention or energy, and do not use any distraction techniques.

Your objective is to sit there and experience the anxiety without resistance.

Stay in this position. Put aside the agenda of urinating and practice allowing the feelings and sensations to rise, peak, and subside on their own. DO NOT TRY TO RELAX OR NEUTRALIZE THE FEELINGS IN ANY WAY. Just observe your anxiety and monitor yourself as the anxiety peaks, and then watch it as it subsides, allowing it to eventually fade.

Carl Robbins explains. Say to yourself, "It's great that I'm feeling anxiety and fear! This is exactly what I need to experience in order to recover! I can embrace/accept/invite my anxiety and simply wait for it to go away on its own. In fact, let's see if I *can intentionally increase it.*" Notice how different this is from *"I must relax."* (Robbins, January 7, 2007).

Build from three minutes. Start with three-minute exposures and, in increasing increments, build up to 15 minutes. If the intensity is so "massive" that you're unwilling to experience your feelings for long, decide *ahead of time* how long you're going to expose yourself to them (it may just be 10 seconds!).

After you've increased the exposure time, try this exercise with higher urgency.

Remember: Doing "Opposite Action" only works if you do it all the way (just going into the restroom if you've been avoiding them is not enough) and with repeated practice. We progress by forming new habits, making them normal. Change your habits, one step at a time.

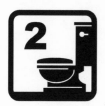 *Out loud with a friend.*

Walk into a bathroom with a friend.

Tell her OUT LOUD that it is taking you a long time and she will have to wait for you.

Two-minute drill with spray bottle.

Sit in a stall for two minutes. Spray a little water in the toilet water to simulate a weak stream.

Repeat every 30 seconds until you are bored.

More desensitizing techniques

Following are some other ways in which you can seek out or provoke your anxiety in non-restroom settings. You are deliberately calling attention to yourself and intensifying the experience of feeling anxious when you:

o Approach someone at an information desk at a mall or the front desk at a hotel and unashamedly say, "I have this problem where I can't urinate around other people, and so I was wondering if you could tell me where I can find the most private, secluded bathroom you know of." Use a "matter of fact" tone and make no attempt to speak softly. Notice his/her reaction; don't just slink away. Optional: Go back and check out what s/he thought when you asked the question (more challenging).

o Go to a drug store or medical supply store and ask if they carry catheters for people with shy bladder syndrome.

o Sit in a hotel lobby, food court, or on public transportation and read Dr. Steven Soifer's book on *"Shy Bladder Syndrome."* Make sure the cover is in plain sight.

Cognitive-Behavioral Therapy has been found to be quite effective in managing the symptoms of paruresis, though it does not appear to be a cure. Some people have reported that using medication and/or various breathing techniques and relaxation methods in tandem with Cognitive-Behavioral Therapy has facilitated their recovery.

Medications

While there are anecdotal reports that a variety of drugs have been used to treat paruresis, there have been no controlled clinical trials to confirm the effectiveness (or lack thereof) of any drug therapies.

Remember, there is no medicine that will cure paruresis. Furthermore, medication alone has not been found to be an effective treatment. Anecdotal reports indicate that the best approach for some may be to combine a drug, such as an SSRI (a category of anti-depressants), with Cognitive-Behavioral Therapy and/or support group work while under a doctor's supervision.

In general, a lot of people deal with constant anxiety, panic attacks, nervousness, shyness, and other common emotional difficulties, such as depression and obsessive-compulsive disorder (OCD). If you have these difficulties, and they are bothering you, it is likely that getting them treated with medication will help you deal with your paruresis.

Many people, like myself, have reported that antidepressants, often in combination with some additional anti-anxiety medicine, make it much easier to work on recovery. But what works for one person may worsen another's condition. This is a complex subject that cannot be properly covered here.

My experience with an anti-depressant

When I began taking an anti-depressant (ostensibly for depression), I found the medication unwittingly helped diminish or alleviate many of my anxiety symptoms that accompanied me whenever I entered a women's restroom. It lowered my level of anxiety, took the "edge" off the persistent rumination I did about bathrooms, reduced my obsessive thoughts, in general, and calmed my mind.

Upon hearing me describe my 40-year battle with paruresis, a psychiatrist chose Prozac™, a common but older Selective Serotonin Reuptake Inhibitor (SSRI), because it seemed to work well on combating obsessive thoughts. Six weeks later, when the drug began to kick in, I felt, "It's okay if I urinate, okay if I don't." It was then that I felt capable of undertaking a CBT program that led to my ultimate recovery.

I like to think of an SSRI as an aid – a big aid. It gives you the presence of mind to put yourself in anxiety-provoking situations so that you can relearn how to function in them and develop a certain distance. By taking the initial edge off the fear we all experience going into a restroom – and keeping you from dwelling on "misfires" – such medication can give you a huge jump start.

The preferred class of drugs prescribed for social anxiety, such as paruresis, is the SSRI because it provides the most benefits with the fewest risks. Besides Prozac™, other common examples are Zoloft™ and Paxil™.

A cautionary note

Although internists and family physicians are allowed to prescribe SSRIs, not all health care professionals are familiar enough with their respective intricacies. To achieve optimum results, I recommend that you consult a psychiatrist, be willing to experiment with different SSRIs, and adjust the dosage until you find the proper amount that works best for you. Anyone on a medication program needs to be carefully monitored by a licensed medical professional.

There are also a large number of medicines known as minor tranquilizers that may be used to treat anxiety and social phobia. Called benzodiazepines (or "benzos" for short), this class of drugs acts to slow down the central nervous system. Common examples include the trade names of Xanax™, Valium™, and Ativan™. Some, but not all, are controlled substances because over time they may cause a physical dependence on the medicine. Usually, though, it is fairly easy to gradually reduce the dose if your doctor agrees that you should no longer take the medicine.

Before you decide to take any medication, it is important to carefully weigh the benefits against the risks. A good discussion of this subject can be found on the IPA's website (www.paruresis.org/drug_faq.htm).

If you are tempted to take medication (particularly if you suffer from depression as well as paruresis), you should discuss all your options in depth with a doctor, preferably a good psychiatrist. In the end only you and your doctor can make the proper decision for you as an individual.

Breathing, Breath-Holding, Relaxation Techniques

In conjunction with the Cognitive-Behavioral Therapy approach, perhaps supplemented by the use of medication, techniques can be taught and practiced to reduce the physical effects of anxiety and to induce relaxation.

Breathing retraining

Deep breathing is a very effective method of relaxation, which is a core component of everything from the "take 10 deep breaths" approach right through to yoga relaxation and Zen meditation. The best way to employ such skills is with the attitude of "If this works, fine. If this doesn't work, that's fine, too."

o Sit in a comfortable position.

o Inhale deeply and slowly through your nose and hold for three seconds.

o Slowly exhale out your mouth.

o Pause momentarily between each deep breath – do no more than three to five deep breaths; otherwise, you may get lightheaded.

Breath-holding

Beginning in early 2005, a technique called "breath holding" has been advocated by some male IPA Discussion Board participants as a means of initiating a urine stream and when used as a complement to Cognitive-Behavioral Therapy. Developed by Monroe Weil, PhD, and described in his article in the May 2001 issue of the *Behavior Therapist*, the method involves inducing relaxation by breath-holding to increase carbon dioxide (CO_2) levels.

In response to my question about the success rate among women, Dr. Weil wrote that "very few individuals have seen me for treatment of paruresis, and all have been men. I feel that the success rate for women should be similar to that of men since the physiological effect of carbon dioxide should be the same" (personal communication, February 2, 2005).

This technique is thought to work because a physical change occurs that causes the external sphincter to relax. As a result of breath-holding, there is an increase in carbon dioxide in the bloodstream and a decrease in oxygen and stress hormones. This practice is well-suited for people who can usually urinate around others once they get a stream going, but have difficulty starting the stream. Here is a brief description from the website of the International Paruresis Association (Levine, n.d.):

o Before attempting to use breath-holding in a restroom, practice holding your breath. If you have respiratory problems, high blood pressure, or any disorder that causes discomfort when holding your breath, first check with your doctor.

Start out holding for 10 seconds, then 15, increasing the time in gradual increments. Pay attention to your body's response to holding your breath.

First get comfortable doing it in a safe setting, such as your home, then practice often in different settings. Only after you are comfortable and calm holding your breath for 45 seconds should you attempt to do so in a restroom in which you are having difficulty starting a stream.

o If the technique is working, you will experience it in a variety of ways. Some describe it as the "pelvic floor dropping" or an unstoppable relaxation of the urinary sphincter muscle. Others say it will make you feel temporarily incontinent.

o Load up on fluids, to the point that your level of urgency is moderate to strong, but not extreme.

o Take your position in the stall, breathe normally, and then exhale (not inhale) about 75% of your breath. Do not take in a big gasp of air before exhaling. You'll have too much oxygen in your lungs, and it will blunt the effect. It's also important to not exhale completely. There needs to be some air left in the lungs.

When holding your breath, pinch your nose if you have to. After about 45 seconds you should experience the pelvic floor "drop," and your stream will start. Once the stream begins, if you start clamping up just exhale again and your stream will return. If your lungs are empty, you may need to take in a small breath and then resume holding it.

o If you find the technique helps you start urinating, with practice it will work at any level of urgency, in every place. Continue practicing and eventually it should be possible to reduce the time required to start urinating. Some people start holding their breath as they approach the restroom so as to cut the time required in a stall accordingly.

o   Some people using the technique report that it works best if a person has a low level of anxiety in the restroom. A period of graduated exposure and support group work may help reduce the level of fear in a public restroom to the point where the breath-holding technique begins to work.

If you are trying it and not getting any results, continue with your recovery program and try it again a few months down the road. The amount of reduction of the tension in the bladder neck and sphincter provided by breath-holding may only be enough to offset a certain level of anxious tension in those areas.

Some additional notes on breath holding from male users:

During the practice period, some people who were afraid to hold their breath for a long time persisted and found that the desired effect on easing urination resulted once they overcame that fear. If you're very concerned, then try holding your breath at a doctor's office where emergency help is available. Most people report they can urinate after around 45 to 60 seconds of breath-holding. That's a long time, but if you are healthy it's not dangerously long.

A cautionary note

Two warnings about using this technique:

1. In some individuals with panic disorder, it has been reported that elevated levels of carbon dioxide can cause symptoms of increased anxiety and panic. If you notice this happening and the symptoms do not improve with practice, then the technique may not be useful for you, or won't become useful unless the panic disorder is treated.

2. If you have any heart condition, check with you doctor before experimenting with the breath-holding method.

Relaxation techniques

Various relaxation methods can help manage stress and reduce anxiety, but should not be the primary intervention for paruresis.

Many Internet sites and books provide detailed information about specific techniques. A good description of some stress management techniques can be located on a website authored by Dr. Susan M. Lark (Lark, n.d.), a foremost authority on women's health issues and the author of nine books. She outlines 14 stress reduction exercises, providing a series of specific steps to help alleviate your symptoms: focusing and meditation, grounding techniques (how to feel more centered), exercises that help you to relax and release muscle tension, visualizations, and affirmations. For further information, go to www.healthy.net/asp/templates/article.asp?PageType=article&ID=1205.

Other links to stress management and emotional wellness:

http://www.optimalhealthconcepts.com/Stress

http://mentalhealth.about.com/od/stress/Stress_Management.htm

Some of the more popular stress reduction techniques are:

o   Progressive Muscular Relaxation (PMR).

o   Massage and other bodywork therapies.

o   Biofeedback.

o   Meditation.

o   Yoga.

Progressive Muscular Relaxation. Progressive relaxation of your muscles reduces pulse rate and blood pressure while decreasing perspiration and respiration rates. Deep muscle relaxation can be used as an anti-anxiety "pill." The body responds to anxiety-producing thoughts and events with muscle tension, which in turn increases the anxiety. Muscle relaxation reduces tension and is incompatible with anxiety. Typically, it involves tensing individual muscle groups for several seconds and releasing the tension – allowing the muscles to relax gradually.

Massage and other bodywork therapies. Recent studies on massage have established that this therapy can lower an individual's blood pressure, induce relaxation, relieve tension, soothe away headaches, loosen tense muscles, or conversely, can be performed to make someone more alert. Massage can help preserve health, heal illness and relieve stiffness and pain. It provides a means to counteract stress and to relax deeply. Massage can be a journey of self-discovery, revealing the pleasure of feeling more at ease and in tune with ourselves.

Biofeedback. Biofeedback is a therapeutic technique using sensitive instruments to measure, amplify, and provide feedback on physiological responses. Various physiological factors of body function and stresses in different parts of the body are fed back to the person in a way that s/he can see and/or hear and ultimately reverse these factors by training various parts of the body to relax.

Meditation. Meditation allows you to create a state of deep relaxation, which is very healing to the entire body. Metabolism slows, as do physiological functions, such as heart rate and blood pressure. Muscle tension decreases. Brain wave patterns shift from the fast beta waves that occur during a normal active day to the slower alpha waves, which appear just before falling asleep or in times of deep relaxation. The idea behind meditation is to consciously relax your body and focus your thoughts on one thing for a sustained period. This occupies your mind, diverting it from the problems that are causing you stress. It gives your body time to relax and recuperate, and to clear away stress hormones that may have built up.

Yoga. Working from the premise that "life is breath, breath is life," yoga places great emphasis on deep, rhythmic, and effective breathing. The principle here is that essential thoughts and messages transmit more effectively when the body is relaxed and the brain is well-oxygenated, helping the body and mind to work more successfully while feeling less tired and less stressed.

Chapter Ten
Taking Action

Take an IPA Workshop

As previously mentioned, IPA workshops are a short-term form of treatment that address cognitive-behavioral approaches to recovery and introduce people to an environment they will experience in a support group. Workshops are thus a good place to begin a treatment program. However, to make a full recovery on a long-term basis, you need to regularly practice the exercises you learn there, in a support group setting, with a "pee buddy," with a trained therapist, or by yourself.

Let me describe for you, in some detail, my first IPA weekend workshop experience.

On a Friday evening, a group of 12 of us, men and women of all ages, met for the first time in a hotel conference room. We went around a table, each of us discussing our own personal struggles with paruresis. I was very nervous when my turn came, worried about comparing my performance to that of others and feeling inferior. However, the sharing of our own experiences helped create safety and trust among participants, and I was very moved upon hearing everyone's stories.

Next we were encouraged to create a behavioral hierarchy, listing our least-feared to our most-feared restroom situations as described in Chapter 9. Our leader explained that most of the following sessions would be devoted to the practice of graduated exposure exercises, in which each person would be paired with a partner (s) to work through his or her hierarchy, one step at a time.

At the start of the morning session, we were instructed to engage in fluid loading to ensure our bladders were moderately full, but not to the point of excess. I was very anxious, since I rarely allowed mine to fill up – typical of the pattern of a lot of paruretics.

As we drank our water in preparation for practice, we were given a set of instructions to follow about how to conduct a practice session (as explained in Step Four, "Begin a practice session," Chapter 9) and also educated about common characteristics of paruretics, current treatment methods for paruresis, and the history and evolution of the IPA.

I was paired with the two other female workshop participants who would become my "pee buddies" for the duration of the workshop. In working with them, I provided direction as to my boundaries, where I wanted them to stand and whether to engage in conversation with each other. I appreciated being in control of my experience.

My comfort threshold allowed me to begin by asking my partners to stand outside my hotel room, positioned at the end of the corridor. I urinated without difficulty and began building on that. Later, in another session, I had them stand directly outside my hotel room. Gradually, throughout the course of the weekend, I brought them closer and closer. For example, I asked one woman to sit on my bed while reading a book (so I knew she was otherwise occupied). By the end of my last session, I felt comfortable urinating with one of them standing at the entrance to the door of my bathroom.

At the end the workshop we had an opportunity to debrief, to share our experiences with each other. We each went around the table, describing the progress we had made and speaking of our goals for the future. It was as if a magical transformation had taken place, the shift of energy palpable. I know I felt like a different person – relaxed, expressive, and talkative – and sensed that same change in others.

We were encouraged to join or start a local support group for paruretics in order to continue practicing graduated exposure exercises, or to practice by ourselves, either with the aid of a trusted "pee buddy" or on our own. Practice was the operative word – each time in different restroom situations, climbing our hierarchies one step at a time.

By the time I enrolled in my second paruresis workshop just one year later, I had made tremendous strides. Three other women also participated, a record number. Now I was ready to attack public restrooms, beginning with the one located in our hotel's lobby and continuing to a shopping center.

My confidence had grown to the point I could easily urinate in a public restroom with others talking, either to one another directly in front of me, or directly to me. By the end of the workshop, I was able to urinate when I instructed one woman to bang on the door to my stall in a public restroom, demanding immediate entrance.

The IPA has run successful workshops strictly for women, which Ruth Lippin, LMSW, and I co-facilitated. Each of the participants, whose ages ranged from 18 through 65, had her own story to tell and benefited from the camaraderie that developed and the opportunity to practice graduated exposure exercises with others. If you are interested in learning more about attending a workshop exclusively for women, write to me at olmert@aol.com.

Disclose Your Condition to Others

Paruresis thrives on secrecy and shame. It's an essential part of recovery to let others know about your paruresis and to observe that most people are supportive and don't view it in the same catastrophic or shameful way that you do. This will help you begin to see that a lot of the shame and guilt you feel don't exist in others; these feelings are self-generated as a consequence of the affliction. Once you tell friends about your paruresis, you'll find that they will be more understanding, and you'll be less nervous around them when the need arises to use a restroom. That alone can reduce anxiety and make it easier to urinate.

Remember to use good sense when choosing with whom you share the fact that you have paruresis. Telling trusted individuals, close friends, and family members is a good way to begin. The benefits to be gained from reaching out to the good people in our lives far outweigh the risks.

Use the Women's IPA Discussion Forum

I established a Discussion Board entitled "Women Only" on the IPA's website in early 2006. A private and "hidden" forum, it is open only to and moderated by women. In order to participate on the "Women Only" Forum, you need to subscribe (it's free):

o Register as a new user on the IPA Talk Forums (www.paruresis.org/phpBB3/) and remember your username. You do not have to use your real name. Use an anonymous username if you are at all concerned about your privacy.

o Once you have created a username, write directly to womensforum@paruresis.org. Ask to have your name added to the "Women Only" Forum and make sure you provide your username. You will be notified by e-mail when this has been completed. (Note: if you already have a username, you still have to supply it so your name can be added).

o After you receive this notification, access the IPA website again. On the left side of your screen, click IPA Talk Forums. Now you will notice that the "Women Only" Forum will automatically appear. You will then have access and can begin to communicate solely with other women.

o By registering as a user, you can also read and post to this and other IPA Forums.

Find a Practice Partner

Now that you've told important people about your condition, ask some of them to be "pee buddies." It does not matter if they are paruretic or not. Don't worry about how you might inconvenience them, or what you owe them in return. That's part of your new behavior of risk taking, right? Friends are committed to helping other friends, and you know you would give up some of your time to assist any one of them if they were in distress, right?

If you are unable to take this step, consider making imaginary "pee buddies" out of your friends. To overcome my fear of entering a restroom with non-paruretic female friends, I made them surrogate "pee buddies" in my mind and without their knowledge. Initially I walked into a large public restroom with a friend, making sure I sat on a toilet at least five stalls apart. I instructed her not to wait for me and gave myself permission to take as long as I needed, even if that meant sitting for quite a while. More often than not, I could urinate, and I congratulated myself after each victory. Over time I moved incrementally closer and closer.

In later sessions, I brought a friend into the restroom and began to engage in casual conversation for the first time in many, many years. Another time, a different friend and I stood in a long line at a movie theater to use one of two available stalls.

Working with a buddy is similar to creating a laboratory out of a bathroom: you two are the guinea pigs and scientists alike. This is great for determining – and pushing – your boundaries, as well as getting used to being around other women while they relieve themselves. You will find that once you get used to your buddy, you will be able to be in much more challenging situations than "in the real world." This is because in a real women's restroom we can't control the situation; we can only deal with it and live in the moment.

Join a Support Group or Create Your Own

Regular participation in a support group is one of the best ways to conquer your fear of urinating in public. With others, you can practice graduated exposure exercises, receive support and encouragement, and discuss your experiences and thoughts during the recovery process.

Support groups are usually free. The process can produce permanent changes in behavior. It is a valuable adjunct for people who are taking medication and/or practicing CBT because group participation happens outside in a real-life setting and serves as a way of increasing the frequency and intensity of work on graduated exposure practice. Supportive partnerships develop in a well-run group that can aid in addressing setbacks and other problems that may crop up in the recovery process. Groups also provide the benefit of working with people who have personal experience in recovering. For a list of current IPA support groups, go to www.shybladder.org/support.php.

It must be emphasized that, up to now, few women have participated in support groups on an ongoing basis. If you're interested in starting one of your own, contact the Shy Bladder Institute (SBI), an IPA auxiliary, at info@shybladder.org. You can find the locations of many of the participants on the IPA Discussion Board by clicking "member list" at http://paruresis.org/phpBB3/. Think about running an ad in a local newspaper or posting a notice on a community bulletin board, either an online forum or at your neighborhood grocery store.

Join the IPA

The International Paruresis Association, Inc. is a nonprofit organization formed in 1996 to help those afflicted with and affected by this form of social anxiety.

For over 10 years, the IPA has consistently worked to:

o Educate the public and the medical establishment on the nature of paruresis.

o Show that paruresis has been one of the most neglected social anxiety disorders and yet afflicts a wide range of people.

o Sponsor workshops to help paruretics overcome this condition.

o Help those afflicted with paruresis overcome the stigma, embarrassment, and isolation associated with it.

o Disseminate the latest information about paruresis.

o Facilitate the establishment of support or self-help groups around the world.

o Expand research to help identify the most clinically effective treatments.

Operated by a small group of professionals and primarily staffed by volunteers, the IPA has already helped thousands of men and women realize a difference in their lives though its workshops, newsletters, websites, counseling sessions, research, and outreach.

The IPA depends on donations to pay for mailings, information packets, administrative help, and other costs. A donor form can be found at http://paruresis.org/join.htm. You can also use this form to let the IPA know how your skills can best be used to educate others about paruresis.

The following stories were written by women who have made remarkable progress in recovering from paruresis. They are very inspirational. Please take the time to read each one.

Best vacation ever

I recently flew from NY to Colorado (with a stop over). Two years ago I would not have considered this trip, at least not without GREAT anxiety. I am still in disbelief that I made this trip with no nervousness at all. From start to finish. I didn't have any misfires. I was able to pee in the airport restrooms (sometimes it took a while) and on the planes (with low urgency). My friend's house was easy, and when we went places, I'd tell her it might take some time. She was fine with it. I was even able to go in the woods a few times, which I always get a kick out of.

What I want people to know most of all is this: Things can get better. I never would have believed this a couple of years ago. This was the most desired trip of my life. The fact that in previous years I would not visit my best friend because of paruresis was sad and frustrating. With encouragement from the IPA, the realization that catheterization use isn't a bad thing if needed, telling others, and desensitizing bit by bit, I have been making continuous progress.

My mom said, "You are cured." This tells me she does not understand the nature of paruresis. I know I'm not cured. I still have many undoable bathroom situations. But I'm getting better.

Getting my life back would not be accurate, because in some respects, I never had one. Paruresis raised such havoc with me that I could never be relaxed for travel or many other things. I feel more like I'm getting a life for the first time at age 46.

A new life

I feel that my life is just now starting. I'll be 49 next month and have just started college. I had actually gone to this same school in 1973, but failed and dropped out due to my paruresis interfering with everything.

Before finding the IPA and learning that many others share my affliction, I lived a life of high anxiety and stress. After telling my friends and family about my problem (plus taking Paxil™), the anxiety has all but disappeared. I've catheterized myself for many years but hate to do it and always wished I could pee like a "normal" person. Now I can pee in many situations without experiencing the heart-pounding terror that used to accompany me in public restrooms.

I recently flew to Salt Lake City, then drove to Yellowstone Park (a five- to six-hour trip). I had to find restrooms along the way, and it was surprisingly easy to pee in a variety of situations. Once I arrived at the park, I had very little trouble using the bathrooms there. Of course, I had brought my catheters along, but only needed to catheterize once in 10 days (when I had waited too long and my bladder was too full to contract properly – a result of many years of holding my urine too long, according to my urologist).

Becoming pregnant for the first time

Several months ago, I posted my abbreviated 'life story' on the main IPA. Thank you to each of you who either replied to my post or e-mailed me privately! That was the start of my recovery, and it also helped me to make one of the most important decisions of my life...whether or not my husband and I should get pregnant.

My very much abbreviated story: Around the age of 21 or so (I am now 32), I was in the bathroom (at college) with a friend of mine. As I sat there in my own, separate stall, I realized that for some strange reason, I was not able to get a flow started. I remember saying out loud, "For heaven's sake, I cannot go!" We laughed, and she said, "Don't worry, that happens to me sometimes... come back in here by yourself in a few minutes." I did, and everything "came out" fine. That was the beginning. No rhyme or reason. No traumatic experience. Everything related to the bathroom and functions therein had been completely normal up until that point.

I don't remember how long it took, but I can remember just a gradual increase in episodes of not being able to go. Unbeknownst to me, at the exact same time, I was also developing what is called interstitial cystitis. I do not know if one caused the other; neither do any of my doctors. IC is a chronic infection of the lining of your bladder... some people are in constant pain. Gratefully, my only symptom currently is that I have to urinate frequently... sometimes twice an hour. Well, as each and every one of you know, that is fine and dandy when you are at home by yourself, but, when out if public... that's when my IC and paruresis really clash!

Things progressively got worse until I reached the point that I could not urinate if my husband was even in the house... he had to go outside and wait in the yard until I gave him the "all clear." That has been, by far, the lowest point in my whole entire life, a point that I never, EVER want to return to.

Well, my urologist decided it was time for some bladder surgery (at that early stage in my IC, I was having quite a bit of pain). It went well, and I am now left with the frequency I told you about previously. I can deal with that any day over pain! Every once in a while, I will have a "flare" of pain, but it is almost always when I have eaten something that obviously does not agree with my IC... very spicy foods, etc.

That surgery took place about seven or so years ago, and my paruresis pretty much stabilized. I gradually built up to where I could "go" with my husband in the same room. Most times, when we are out, I can go if the restroom is empty. Every once in a great while, I can go if others are in the room, but it has to be pretty noisy and crowded (with no one in the stall right beside me). My husband is my rock and my foundation. He has been with me for 14 years now and has been there every step of the way. He is my true hero!

Now, to my big news. My husband and I talked, and talked, and talked some more. And we decided several months ago, that after almost 14 years of marriage, paruresis or not, we were going to try to start a family. I posted for the very first time on the IPA website and received several wonderful responses from people. Thank you to each of you who inspired me to take this tremendous leap of faith! Well, after a couple of months of "really" trying (you know, marking your calendar, circling your ovulation dates, getting the go ahead from your OB-GYN), I am very happy to announce that sometime around November 20, there will be a new addition to our family!!!! We are SOOOO excited!

On top of the normal "what ifs" and anxieties, I have this whole paruresis issue, but I'm dealing with that. My OB-GYN knows about it. In fact, I took Steven Soifer's book with me on my first visit. She was very understanding. She knew nothing of the subject, but was understanding.

So, here I am. My very first pregnancy! I just wanted to share this news with the few people on this earth who will completely understand all of my excitement, worry, elation, fears, and anticipation. Please, please, I would LOVE any comments and especially ANY advice on how to deal with these coming months. You know, the constant urine samples, the sudden urges to go at the mall, etc. I will welcome any advice and words of encouragement!

I see progress in every aspect of my pee problem and my life

Since October I have been addressing my paruresis problem, and I am beginning to look back on how much progress I have made. I am 37 years old. I hope my story can help someone. I started desensitization work with a phobia therapist in NY recommended by Steven Soifer. This work included me bringing two of my best girlfriends on separate visits to the sessions with me to see exactly how I struggle and to get me over the embarrassment of it all. I also told other close friends to take away the stigma in my head of having paruresis. I told my boyfriend who seemed to understand. After all, people really don't think it's such a bad thing when you tell them.

And since I think we all (paruretics) have personal issues that contribute to our feelings of no control over our bodies and our problem, I dealt with those that, for me, send me over the edge, mine being my family issues. I changed my job to a less stressful one. I made my pee problem my sole focus for the last six months. Just this week my therapist said that I could probably stop seeing her regarding my pee problem if I wanted to. I still have a few challenging situations that I would like to explore with her. The important thing is that I have developed a support system outside of my therapist, that I no longer feel isolated in my problem and that I see progress in every aspect of my pee problem and my life.

Changing perceptions and perspective about "what others think" propelled me forward

I am 44 years old, living in Southern Dutchess County in New York State. I have had paruresis since I was around 11 or 12. I would call it a moderate case since I could always pee in a private lockable restroom; public restrooms were the problem for me.

I have, in the last six months or so, made such progress with my battle with paruresis that I think it is over, or nearly so. One of my biggest problems was in a "two-seater." I had been having success in bigger bathrooms with lots of stalls and could pee if the adjacent stalls were empty. I think that restrooms with no outside door still are a bit of an issue for me (like those in theaters or other public places that tend to develop long lines). I can now pee 100% of the time in the "two-seater" at work with someone in the next stall and/or at the sink and/or with conversations happening all around me. Not sure, though, if I can participate in those conversations yet, but anything is possible.

I attribute my success to a change in my perceptions and perspective. I really believe that no one cares how long it takes me to pee or that I'm peeing at all. I came to realize that "regular" people sometimes take a few seconds to get going. I stopped caring what others might think and I really surprised myself the first time I was able to pee in the two-seater at work with someone sitting on the couch near the entrance. I walked out of there on cloud nine since I had done something I never imagined I could or would do. That success led to a bit of confidence (or at least a feeling that trying might lead to another success) and that led to more successes and more confidence, and the monster lost its size.

I was suicidal over the humiliation I felt at one point; now I've recovered

I'm from Philadelphia, and I am 49 years old today! I have had paruresis since I was a child, about eight years old. My case has improved over the years from fairly severe in my 20s to mild today. I attribute my progress to a number of factors, one of which was childbirth at the age of 37, which seemed to "loosen things up" (and also gave me stress incontinence, which is a VERY minor nuisance compared to paruresis.)

Other things which helped me were going on Paxil™ for social anxiety, and some determined desensitization work on my own. I can usually void anywhere now except very quiet public restrooms with only one other person. I still have much more difficulty with people I know than with strangers, though I can now go with my partner in the bathroom with me! Interestingly, I never had many problems on planes or other moving vehicles because of the privacy of the toilets and the extensive background noise. For me it has always been the fear of someone hearing me, or waiting for me, that has driven my paruresis. I have never used a catheter but would gladly have done so in my younger years; paruresis constricted my life to an extreme at one point, almost destroying me socially, personally and professionally. I was suicidal over the humiliation I felt.

1. Understand that paruresis is a type of social anxiety. Read and absorb introductory information about it at www.paruresis.org/about_avoidant_paruresis.htm. Continue reading the "Best of the Boards," "Links" and "Information/ Resources" sections on the IPA Home Page (www.paruresis.org). As you've seen, there are more similarities than differences between female and male paruretic sufferers.

2. Realize that most people have trouble urinating from time to time. But one who truly suffers from paruresis feels intense anguish about going to the bathroom when others are around; their normal daily function is impaired to one degree or another.

3. Rule out the possibility you have a physical impediment or medical cause by consulting with a health care professional. Though it is unlikely, you may have a physical rather than a psychological condition. Be sure to consult a physician if you suspect that may be the case, but remember some are ignorant about paruresis. You may have to educate them, so bring along some materials from the IPA Home Page (or use the information in Appendix 4).

4. Keep up with educational materials. Make sure you understand what paruresis is and isn't and the methods that have been most effective in treating this condition. For starters, obtain a copy of *Shy Bladder Syndrome: Your Step-by-Step Guide to Overcoming Paruresis.*

5. Read posts on the IPA Discussion Board at www.parureis.org (another good website is www.paruretic.com). While males participate more often than women, you will learn much, make a connection to fellow paruretic sufferers, and develop empathy for those in your situation. As you become more comfortable, consider responding to a post, or, better yet, submit your own query. If you have privacy issues, you can use an alias.

6. **Learn about issues unique to female paruretics** and join the Women's Forum on the IPA Discussion Board. Locate the special section on the IPA website called "Women's Resources" at www.paruresis.org and join the Women's Forum on the IPA Discussion Board by e-mailing womensforum@paruresis.org. Reach out to and support other female paruretics in their journey toward recovery. They will relate to and understand the mental (and physical) pain you are experiencing.

7. **Remember that secrets are poison.** Tell important people in your life about your paruresis, particularly those you're close to. A very important step is to write about your problem, open up to your spouse or significant other about it, tell a parent if you have one that will be sympathetic, tell a very close trusted friend, a clergyperson, and/or your primary care doctor (but be prepared for the possibility of having to educate others).

8. **Learn to catheterize yourself** because it is the ultimate back-up plan for those times when you simply cannot urinate (think of it as a "get out of jail free" card in Monopoly). Before doing so, first consult with an internist, a nurse, nurse practitioner, or a specialist, such as a urologist or OB/GYN. If possible, seek out a female. Be prepared for the possibility that you may have to make them aware of the condition. Do not take NO for an answer and continue your quest to find someone who can teach you the procedure.

9. **Recognize that there is no instant "cure,"** no super hypnotic suggestion, and no magic pill or potion you can swallow to make your symptoms disappear. Rather plan to commit to undergoing a treatment program based on Cognitive-Behavioral Therapy. This method allows you to recover slowly and gradually, and it can be used in conjunction with medications and other adjunct therapies and techniques, such as relaxation methods and breath-holding. I can't over emphasize that you have to really, really want to recover – enough so that you will do anything and everything it takes to achieve your goals.

10. **Consider taking medications** that might allow you to begin a recovery program under a doctor's supervision. Anti-depressants (SSRIs), such as Prozac™ or Paxil™, may work for some but not all to diminish your level of anxiety, reduce obsessive thoughts, and calm your mind to the point that you can fully undertake a recovery program. While it may take about five to six weeks for the medications to kick in, some paruretics have found they take the "edge" off the fear they experience upon entering a restroom, prevent them from dwelling on 'misfires' or constantly ruminating about bathrooms.

11. **Become aware of other "tools" that may facilitate the urination process**, e.g., *Stadium Gal*™, *TravelMate*™. (See separate section on "Other Options When You Can't Urinate in a Restroom" in Appendix 1).

12. **Attend at least one IPA workshop.** For many, this experience is magical and transformational. In a small group setting, you will have the opportunity to meet and discuss your particular symptoms and avoidance patterns, learn about and practice desensitization exercises with others, begin to change your thought patterns, and much, much more. Workshop attendees report that behavior modification brings about changes in cognitive thinking (rational/irrational). It works the other way around, too: dealing with the irrationality helps to improve or alter the behavior. Yes, you can make progress on your own but probably will improve faster by attending a workshop – they offer intangibles and insights that you may not otherwise achieve. Check http://www.shybladder.org/workshops.php for a workshop schedule.

13. **PRACTICE, PRACTICE, PRACTICE graduated exposure exercises on a regular basis.** Learn how it works so that it WILL work. Create a written hierarchy, a list of increasingly challenging situations. Apply graduated exposure to your hierarchy list and begin to practice, either by yourself, with a "buddy," and/or a trained therapist. While helpful, it is not necessarily essential to practice with a partner who has paruresis.

Once you are totally familiar with the technique, you can ask a female friend or spouse/significant other – someone with whom you're very comfortable – to be your practice "mate" in terms of accompanying you to a bathroom. Or, for that matter, you can make an "imaginary pee buddy" out of a female friend without even disclosing your condition to her.

The key and operative words here are *practice* and *reinforcement* – you must practice often and diligently in order to accelerate your progress. You will not get better if you never venture into a public restroom. So visit restrooms at every opportunity, even if you can't go and only want to wash your hands. Accept that the more frequently you practice, the sooner you'll see results. Look for the most challenge you're capable of handling, not just the "safe choice." Schedule regular practice sessions and combine them with incidental trips to the supermarket or library. Ensure that you have water bottles all over the place at home, work, restaurants, and even at church or synagogue. Drink up! More than anything else, ongoing persistent and consistent practice will allow you to overcome or recover from your paruresis in a timely manner.

14. **Attend IPA support group meetings**. Once you complete a workshop – or perhaps before you enroll in one – consider joining a support group if one exists in your area. Fellow sufferers understand how debilitating this disorder is. Here you will receive a lot of emotional support and the opportunity to practice desensitization exercises with a partner on a regular basis. If a support group doesn't exist in your area, think about starting one on your own.

15. **Maintain a positive, determined, and focused attitude**. Find something good about every try, and remember that there's no such thing as "failure" – a misfire means that you are 15 minutes away from urinating! Focus on your progress. Look at the long range goal. Recognize that by actively confronting your fears, you will have the opportunity to lead a full and productive life without this problem. Change is possible – even if it is slow or occasional. You need to be your own best friend.

16. **Attend follow-up workshops** in order to relive and expand the gains made in your recovery.

17. **Don't be afraid to take some risks.** Face your thoughts and fears, experience the anxiety, and find out that you didn't die from them; in time the anxiety will decrease.

18. **Keep a three ring binder, online "scrapbook," or journal** of "good" postings, success stories, positive self-talk, e.g., "I can urinate when there are people around," and other information about paruresis. Put a lot of detail into it, the triggers, how you felt, who was there, where they were, echo level of the restroom, layout, type of people present, and the outcomes. Track your progress over time, and you will begin to notice a gradual pattern of overall improvement.

19. **For long airplane flights, consider the prudent use of** Desmopressin Acetate (DDAVP™, Stimate™, Minirin™), a medication available in tablet or nasal spray form that is prescribed to increase urine concentration and decrease urine production. Normally, it is used to prevent nocturnal enuresis (bed wetting), but it has been found to be helpful to some paruretics.

20. Learn some valuable lessons on the path to recovery that may carry over to other aspects of your life:

> o *People do not pay attention to your bathroom habits,* how long you're taking, whether you are making noise, etc., contrary to many people's life-long beliefs. We only think they do because we are hyper-focused on bathrooms.

> o *Cultivate what can be called a relaxed, "ho-hum attitude"* – it's fine if I urinate, fine if I don't. Give up your attachment to the results. Once you begin to climb your hierarchy and are gradually achieving more "successes" than misfires, just keep practicing and continue to give yourself a pat on the back for each attempt. Reward yourself for practice. If you can't void, do not beat yourself up but rather repeat the previous stage when you were able to urinate.

o *Give yourself permission* to spend as much time as you want in a stall. You have that *entitlement*. Dr. Howard Liebgold, a physician who serves as a facilitator and advisor to the IPA, strongly emphasizes that point. Dr. Soifer refers to this concept as "staking your territory," and it is an important one to grasp and put into practice.

o *Make a game out of your recovery or consider it an adventure.* You know you are winning the game when you stand by the entrance of a restroom waiting in anticipation for, if not looking forward to, someone else to walk in so you can follow them.

o *Be good to yourself.* If you suffer from "performance anxiety" issues, like so many of us, you are probably extra hard on yourself. Learn to stop putting a lot of pressure on yourself, to lower your self-expectations, and to stop – to the fullest extent possible – being performance-driven.

o *Avoidance exacts a high price.* There is nothing better to control anxiety and embarrassment than avoidance and fleeing (in the short term). But the problem is, it has side effects – you don't have a life.

o *Become pro-active, not complacent.*

21. **Fully document your case of paruresis with a physician.** If you are ever in the position of being forced to produce a urine specimen, at least there will be a paper trail of your existing condition.

22. **Learn to drink more fluids on a regular basis.** Many of us are habitually used to refraining from drinking liquids to avoid having to urinate. While it is not necessary to follow the "8-10 glasses of water per day" rule of thumb, it is important to keep your body hydrated. Make a conscious effort to do some of the following: take a water break frequently throughout the day; take a sip when you pass a water fountain; carry a bottle of water with you in your car; start a meal with a cup of soup; drink a beverage with each meal; and drink more when exercising, especially if it's hot or humid.

23. **Join and donate to the IPA,** the only organization of its kind that works for you. Membership information can be found online at www.paruresis.org/join.htm or by calling 1-800-247-3864.

24. **Take social action.** Before or after your recovery, take action in changing the conditions that may contribute to paruresis in the first place. Consider going public about your condition, making others aware. Educate a physician or nurse on the nature and effect of paruresis and disseminate the latest information about it. Speak with school officials about inadequate toilets, the problems with drug testing of students, and bullying. Advocate for the rights of people with paruresis who have been unfairly discriminated against in drug testing.

Expand research to help identify the most clinically effective treatments. At your work place, health club or other public facility, if you find a particular restroom design objectionable, let the management know and ask them to do something about it. Go into a store, ask to use a restroom, and make a minor fuss if refused or if the conditions are terrible.

Campaign for the passage of "potty parity" laws in your state and municipality in order to increase the ratio of women's toilets to men's. Become an advocate for greater availability and accessibility to public restrooms and better design for people with shy bladders, e.g., floor-to-ceiling partitions, which are common throughout Europe.

Do something – don't just sit quietly waiting for others to take action. Use your mouth, intellect, phone, and computer skills to agitate for the changes we need. You are likely to feel more empowered in relation to paruresis as a result.

25. **Don't ever give up or give in.** Keep the faith that you can and will recover from paruresis – trust the process. See every day as a day of opportunity and every time you have to go as an opportunity. Set yourself small, reachable goals and reward yourself mentally or tangibly. Accept that the path may involve two steps forward and one step back – but ultimately will lead to recovery.

Appendices

Appendix 1:
Other Options When You Can't Urinate in a Restroom

Appendix 2:
Design of Women's Restrooms and Toilet Facilities

Appendix 3:
More about the Author's Experience with Paruresis

Appendix 4:
Useful Information about Paruresis to Bring
with You to a Health Care Professional

Chapter 8 mentions the availability of various assistive techniques and devices that may be of use to women seeking alternatives to using a public restroom. They include:

o Urinary collection bags.

o Disposable urinal bags.

o Urinating while standing up (with or without the aid of a funnel).

o Female and portable urinals.

o Portable toilets and privacy tents.

The following section explores each of these techniques and devices in some depth.

Urinary Collection Bags

External collection devices funnel urine via a pouch to a collection container for disposal. These flexible pouches stick, by adhesive straps or suction, to the outside of the labia, preventing urine from leaking around the device. The end of the pouch connects to a larger drainage bag. The bag is worn around the thigh or calf, thus allowing freedom of movement, and is emptied periodically.

These devices are typically used for females afflicted with chronic or severe incontinence. According to a few research studies, they are less successful in containing urine than some of their male counterparts, such as condom catheters (Angelo, 2002).

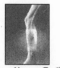

The Stadium Gal™

Reprinted with permission
of BioRelief.com

One example of an external collection device is *The Stadium Gal for Women*™, a female urinary pouch that can be completely hidden beneath loose-fitting jeans or pants and is, therefore, totally discrete.

The pouch is non-latex and contains an odor-barrier pouch film. The collection bag is attached to the inner calf by means of elastic straps than can be cut down to fit your leg. At the bottom of the pouch is a convenience drain that connects to the leg bag system.

Emptying the *Stadium Gal*™ is done by placing one's foot on the rim of a toilet bowl and opening the T-tap valve. The *Stadium Gal*™ can be worn up to 24 hours, and the collection bag holds 1000 ml or about 34 oz. You can find it at www.biorelief.com/store/stadiumgal.html#.

A similar system, manufactured by the Hollister Corporation, consists of a form-fitting cup held in place by the labia and panties; it connects with a line leading to a collection bag so a woman can move around freely (www.athomemedical.com/Absorbent-Pouches/Hollister-Female-Urinary-Pouch.asp).

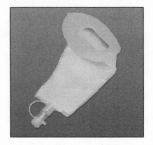

Reprinted with permission of BioRelief.com

Disposable Urinal Bags

These devices consists of a portable "bag within a bag" system for urination while on the go or in less than desirable situations. Basically one urinates into this pouch, and there is a substance inside – a mixture of bioactive polymers and enzymes – that absorbs the liquid, makes it gel instantly, and also deodorizes. When "done," the pouch is spill-proof and, because it is waste-disposal safe, it can be thrown away after use. The bag is also non-toxic, small, lightweight, and inexpensive.

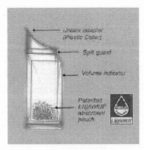

TravelJohn™

Reprinted with permission of Reach Global Industries Inc.

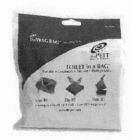

Restop 1™

Reprinted with permission of American Innotek Inc.

The *TravelJohn*™ and *The WAG BAG*® *Toilet in a Bag*™ Disposable Urine Bags are two examples of these products (http://www.traveljohn.com/ or http://thepett.com/).

Urinating while Standing Up

In much earlier times, women customarily urinated while standing up, and this practice still continues today in many undeveloped countries.

In ancient Egypt, men squatted and women stood to urinate. In the 19th Century, Apache Indian men would usually squat while the women would relieve themselves standing up. In Japan, the high society ladies of 19th Century Kyoto perfected the art of passing urine into a bucket while standing upright (Research Pod, n.d.).

Less than 100 years ago, when outhouses were still the norm, our female ancestors had to choose between standing to urinate or sitting on a toilet seat that was below freezing. In cold climates, squatting could be hazardous if the body made contact with ice or frozen ground. Understandably, many women not only chose to stand, but designed their clothing (such as skirts and underwear) to make this easier by adding placket openings.

Today in less developed Third World countries, women are still urinating standing up, and this technique for urinating is considered normal. Many women often wear a sarong and no underwear. One also can see evidence of women standing up in the rural countrysides of many nations. In Africa, even signs forbidding public urination often show a picture of a woman urinating while standing (http://www.bigfoto.com/africa/ghana/ghana-66.jpg).

Most likely, the majority of women doubt it is even possible for them to urinate in a standing posture without soiling their clothes. This is particularly true for those of us living in western societies.

Physiologically, women are able to urinate standing up in a way similar to that of men. This may be done by manipulating the genitalia in a certain way, orienting the pelvis at an angle and rapidly forcing the urine stream out. An alternative method is to use a tool, as described below, to assist in the process.

A female urination device or aid is a small funnel that enables a woman to urinate while standing upright. Before about 1997 few such devices appear to have been widely available. Interestingly, a similar tool was patented back as far as 1918. That model, the "Sanitary Protector" by Edyth Lacy, specifies a "cheap device ... [to be] used but once, being especially suitable as a sanitary device in public toilet rooms." She notes that it is "accordingly unnecessary for the user to sit upon the closet seat; and the urine is led off without danger of soiling the clothes of the user or the closet." It was to be "made of a cheap readily destructible material, such as stiff paper, which can be readily disposed of after its use." A similar device was patented in 1956 and others followed, each designed to prevent a woman from making contact with a toilet seat ("female urination device", 2007).

Attitudes toward urinating while standing have begun to change, particularly among younger women. As evidence, a book has even been published on the subject. Called *How to Pee Standing Up: Tips for Hip Chicks*, it is written by Anna Skinner and is more of an entertaining survival guide, teaching younger women how to function in an independent way.

Recently, a number of non-invasive assistive devices have been brought to market to facilitate urination while standing. They allow a woman to pull down her pants and squat, or with practice, to void through the open zipper of her jeans as conveniently as a man. When held securely under the crotch, and with underpants pushed to the side, these devices direct urine away from the body into a suitable place, such as a toilet or a container.

For those interested, I've identified several websites that offer information on the topic of using assistive devices as an aid to urination.

www.freshette.com

www.goyourway.net or
www.pmateusa.com

www.mysweetpee.com

www.travelmateinfo.com

www.urinelle.biz

www.whizaway.com

www.whizzy4you.com

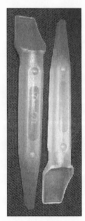

TravelMate™

Reprinted with
permission of
Travel Mate

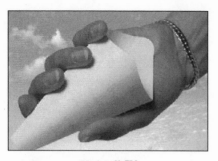

Urinelle™

Arte Viva (AV)

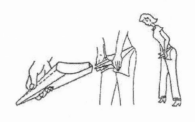

P-Mate™

Reprinted with permission
of Karen Diamond

Female and Portable Urinals

Along with chamber pots (used domestically or privately) and *bourdalou* (likely to have been used by women publicly), female urinals made of glass or pottery have actually been around for centuries, long before water closets were ever invented. Popular in the early part of the 18th Century, many were remarkably beautiful (Penner, June 2005).

Today, improved portable devices that substitute for a regular toilet can be very helpful for those who have difficulty using a public restroom. This type of urinal consists of a hand-held container that is lightweight, solid, and easy to use. While the majority are used in lieu of bedpans and/or for partially immobilized people, a few have recently been introduced that permit portability and can be used while traveling in a car, boat, or when camping or skiing.

The Feminal® is a female urinal designed and developed by Linda Asta, a female urology nurse-entrepreneur. She is also the inventor of *Asta-Cath*®, the plastic device that allows a woman to easily locate the entrance to her urethra. (See the section on "Catheterization – Finding Immediate Relief" in Chapter 8). *The Feminal*® has a smooth, ergonomic shape and consists of a flat base and a lip that is pressed up against the vulva, creating a seal to contain the urine. It is available on-line at www.brucemedical.com/femfemur.html or www.valuemedicalsupplies.com/feminal.htm, or through medical supply firms.

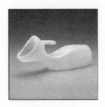

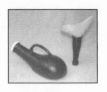

The Feminal®

The Millie®

The Lady J® connected to **Little John®**

Reprinted with permission
of Linda Asta, RN,
A+ Medical Products

Reprinted with permission
of Viscot Medical LLC
© Viscot Medical LLC 2000

Reprinted with permission
of Gaylen Brotherson,
MBA Holdings, Inc.

The Millie® is a female urinal designed with a special shape for women. It holds up to one liter with volume markings on the side and is available through medical supply companies or online at www.valuemedicalsupplies.com/millie.htm.

The Lady J Adapter® is an anatomically designed funnel which snaps into place on the *Little John®* portable urinal. Made of unbreakable plastic, the container can hold up to 32 ounces and is available online at http://www.cabelas.com/spod-1/0014250.shtml.

Portable Toilets and Privacy Tents

Portable toilets and privacy tents may provide an alternative for those who seek peace and quiet when they want to urinate, especially in outdoor situations. These products are available online or through camping goods stores. Some paruretics have reported good results with using such devices when they travel by car or participate in outdoor recreational activities. Here are four examples of portable toilets:

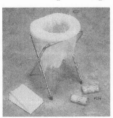

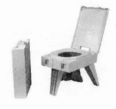

Stansport® Folding Portable Toilet

The PETT® Toilet

Reprinted with permission
of Stansport, Inc.
www.epcamps.com/portable_toilet.html

Reprinted with permission
of Phillips Environmental Products
www.thepett.com

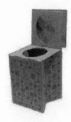

**A portable toilet made of
corrugated paper board**

Reprinted with permission
of GT Products LLC
http://www.chemisan.com/product.html

*Inflate-A-Potty
Portable® Sanitary Toilet*

Reprinted with permission
of Brite Times, Inc.
http://potties.com/adult.htm

Here are four examples of privacy tents:

The PUP™ Privacy Shelter

Reprinted with permission
of Phillips Environmental Products, Inc.
www.thepett.com

Restop™ Privacy Tent

Reprinted with permission
of American Innotek, Inc.
www.restop.com

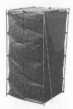

Stanisport ®

Reprinted with permission
of Stansport, Inc.

www.safetycentral.com

TravelJohn™ Privacy Shelter

Reprinted with permission
of Reach Global Industries, Inc.

www.traveljohn.com

A Brief History of Toilet Design

Toilet design has changed little in about 150 years

The history of public toilets is scarce, and, in fact, there is a great deal of controversy surrounding who was responsible for the invention of the toilet. The oldest working toilet with "flushing" water is said to be in the Minoan Palace at Knossos on the Greek island of Crete and is thought to be about 4,000 years old ("History of plumbing", n.d.).

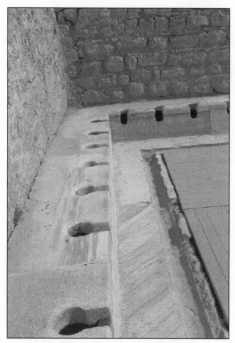

Several of the more advanced ancient civilizations, Greek, Indian and Roman, dating back to about 2600 B.C.E., had a system providing running water to citizens in the larger cities. Used by the local populace and by travelers alike, these facilities were largely communal.

The Romans, in particular, found public toilets important, but they were discontinued when the empire declined.

Ancient Roman latrines

Source: Wikipedia Commons
in the public domain

Credit for the invention of the forerunner to the modern flush toilet is usually bestowed on Sir John Harrington, a godson of Queen Elizabeth I, as far back as 1596. His design of the "water closet" was not taken seriously in England but was adopted in France under the name *Angrez* ("Flush Toilet", n.d.).

Others claim Sir John's idea was not widely adopted because there was no supply of running water to flush it ("Toilet History", n.d.). In any case, the English public remained faithful to the chamber pot.

Approximately 200 years later, in 1775, English watchmaker Alexander Cummings made improvements by putting a water trap under the bowl. Many consider this design as the first modern flushing toilet. Building on his concepts, four British entrepreneurs – George Jennings, Thomas Crapper, Joseph Bramah, and Thomas Twyford – and other inventors took the toilet into the next century. The most essential attributes proved to be the washdown pipe design, a siphon attached to the bowl (in order to keep foul odors from issuing out of the sewer), and a reliable valve or siphon in the tank so as to enable a rapid first flush followed by a slower after-flush.

It was only in Victorian times that public toilets appeared in any large numbers. The Public Health Act of 1848 – legislating on the sanitary conditions of England and Wales and considered "one of the great milestones in public health history" – called for "Public Necessaries" to be provided to improve sanitation.

In 1852, the engineer George Jennings invented an improved flushing system and popularized public lavatories by installing them in the Crystal Palace for the Great Exhibition of 1851 in London. More than 800,000 visitors paid one penny each to use them. These toilets were hailed as a great success and led to an acknowledgement of the "necessity of making similar provisions for the public whenever large numbers are congregated [to alleviate] the sufferings which must be endured by all, but more especially by females on account of the want of them" (Penner, 2005).

The Great Exhibition could be said to have marked the start of a more civilized era in women's facilities. On the other hand, the model of the ladies' room that was established – private stalls each with toilet, lock, and door – became the dominant one that still remains in use today (Penner, 2005).

In the 1880s, toilets that could be used by either gender began to appear. Still, nearly all public conveniences were for men, with few supplied for women. The logic was that far more men were away from home than women, either for work or leisure.

In Victorian times it was assumed that "respectable" women did not go to work and did not travel around cities or visit places of entertainment. Urinals were also cheaper to construct. The British writer George Bernard Shaw campaigned for facilities for women, but he was battling against the feeling that it was somehow not decent to have public toilets for women ("Stoke-on-Trent", n.d.).

There were a number of small-scale experiments to provide women with alternate accommodation. In London, around 1898, "urinettes" were first installed on a trial basis in one female public lavatory. Narrower than conventional water closets with curtains instead of doors, they were expected to "answer much the same purpose as urinals in the men's section," (Penner, 2005) that is, they were to be used for relieving oneself quickly. On the face of it, urinettes appeared viable. They were perceived to be more space-efficient than water closets, and they were also cheap – only a halfpenny was to be charged for their use instead of the usual penny. At that time, women wore skirts with underclothing typically open at the crotch so that they could relieve themselves easily, without having to pull down their drawers.

The early urinettes were used, more or less, when the stalls were busy or by women lacking proper change for the door lock. However, there was a type fitted in Portsmouth, England at the turn of the century that was only a few inches from the floor, with instructions to urinate standing. The idea probably so frightened women that they were hardly ever used! (Crimson, 1998).

Back home in America, early settlers, like their Native American counterparts, used rivers, woods, and shrubs to fulfill their toilet needs. In 1857, the first American patent for a toilet, the "plunger closet," was granted, though on the U.S. plains, the outhouse still predominated. It was a small building constructed over an open pit with a bench inside into which several holes were fashioned (sometimes it was a multi-seater, and the whole family would often go at once).

Chamber pots were still in use by the masses although the wealthy had flush toilets imported from England. These pots varied from open buckets to decorative ceramic containers with tight fitting lids and were emptied daily either into the street or an outhouse.

Largely unsuccessful improvements continued to be made in the 1870s to 1890s in the search for a sanitary "water closet" (Odell, 1997). American designs were considered generally inferior to English ones, and most "water closets" of this period were imported.

At the end of the 19th Century, public restrooms were beginning to become an accepted fact in the large cities of Europe and the United States. However, in rural areas as in the poorer section of cities, the outhouse was used well into the 20th Century – and still is in rural Alaska.

So, although the modern flush toilet as we know it was invented about 150 years ago, the design of public toilet stalls in America remains fundamentally unchanged. For years, the primary goal of architects and builders seemed to be to squeeze as much utility as possible out of the least amount of space, often with the least amount of money.

Bathroom users' needs seldom considered

Until relatively recently, very little consideration was given to the needs – physiological psychological, cultural, social – and priorities of bathroom users. Alexander Kira, Professor Emeritus of Architecture at Cornell University, was one of the first to try to turn the tide. In his groundbreaking book, *The Bathroom* (first published in 1966, and revised in 1976), he studied both men and women's behavioral, psychological, and sociological responses to the "bathroom experience" and how the experiences differ from public to private environments. Out of this research came the notion that while economy and efficient construction are still important considerations, so too are the specific requirements and preferences of the people who use the bathroom.

The needs of female bathroom users, among others, have seldom been taken into account. However, two university professors, Kathryn Anthony and Clara Greed, are beginning to make their voices heard as strong advocates for improved restroom design. Both have researched, published, and lectured extensively on the subject of inadequate public toilet provision for women.

Kathryn Anthony, a Professor of Architecture at the University of Illinois at Urbana-Champaign and a noted expert on toilet design, explains the reasons why the female population has been ignored:

> Historically speaking, architects, contractors, engineers, and building code officials rarely contacted women to learn about their special restroom needs, and, until recently, women were rarely employed in these male-dominated professions or in a position to

be able to effect change. Even today, these professions remain male-dominated (Anthony and Dufresne, 2007, p. 268).

Clara Greed, a professor who specializes in "inclusive urban planning" at the University of the West of England and the author of *Inclusive Urban Design*, concurs that womens' needs are not always recognized by planners, and few women are themselves in government, even at the local level.

Undoubtedly the cultural attitudes and gender composition of those responsible for setting these standards (for public toilet provision) is a key factor explaining the lack of progress. Many of the regulations and standards governing toilet provision are the result of deliberations of nominated, unrepresentative committees. The lack of women particularly in senior positions is an enduring issue in the world of town planning and urban governance but the problem is even more extreme in the world of sanitary engineering, especially at the local authority level (Greed, 2003).

The Americans with Disabilities Act (ADA), which officially took effect in 1992, resulted in some major changes in the architectural design and layout of washroom facilities but did not go far enough. The law mandated that all washrooms, whether they're newly constructed or renovated, must be usable by people with disabilities. However, even the disabled segment of the population is a very diverse group in terms both of age and of the severity and nature of the disabling condition or conditions involved. So even after the implementation of the ADA, the lack of standardization within the design and fitting of the accessible toilet has meant that many disabled people must "make do" with the level of provision that is currently offered. "Nonetheless, although the ADA succeeded in providing greater *accessibility* for persons with disabilities in public restrooms, the problem of *availability* remains," wrote Anthony (Anthony, 2007, p. 270).

Today's design standards do not fully recognize, represent, and include the views of many segments of the population. Among them are the elderly, the obese, families with infants and young children, pregnant, menstruating, and breast-feeding women, those with invisible physical disabilities, those who are opposite-gender caregivers, those who have either intermittent or chronic medical conditions that cause them to frequently need to use a bathroom – and those of us who are "restroom-challenged" paruretics.

Public toilets in the United States reflect poor design, especially relative to European ones. They typically have open seams in the partitions with big openings above and below. The standard design for toilet compartments is side panels and a door that start 12 inches above the floor and reach 60 inches above the finished floor with about a half-inch gap between the door and the stall. By contrast, European public bathroom stalls are frequently fully enclosed, with full doors and floor-to-ceiling partitions.

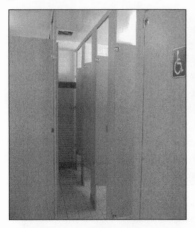 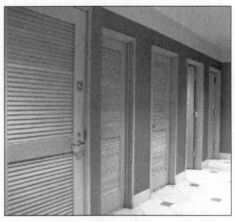

Standard women's bathroom; movie theater in San Francisco

Ideal USA bathroom such as those found in Europe; Nordstrom's in San Francisco

Photos by Carol Olmert

As we've seen, there are many degrees of paruresis. With improved design standards, it is possible that a man with a mild form might be able to use a public bathroom if there were partitions between urinals. For a woman with paruresis, having a stall with walls and doors that reach from the ceiling to the floor might mean the difference between her being able to use the facility or not. It is clear that both genders would benefit from having more personal space and private territory in public restrooms.

On some fronts, there is good news. Family restrooms are increasing in number – at airports, shopping malls, and sports facilities. Unisex facilities are becoming more available, particularly at college and university campuses, in urban nightclubs, and in public parks. More laws are being passed to increase the number of fixtures for women, as well as for men. New technology advances, such as the installation of automatic faucets, flushers, soap and paper towel dispensers, cleaning systems, and other touch-free devices in restrooms, have resulted in improved sanitation.

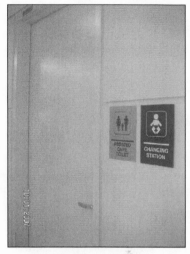

**Family restroom,
Midway Airport, Chicago**

Photo by Carol Olmert

But progress is slow. According to Kathryn Anthony, "These trends are still by far the exception rather than the rule, and the United States continues to lag far behind other countries when it comes to the availability of public restrooms. In most American cities, finding a public restroom is still a challenge, and the (2006 World Toilet Forum in Bangkok, Thailand) theme, 'happy toilet, healthy life' remains an ideal and not yet a reality" (Anthony, 2006).

Many public facilities, particularly in major U.S. cities, have increasingly fallen into a state of disrepair, have limited hours of operation, or been closed by local governments who cite crime or cost. Sometimes community groups organize to oppose their installation. They are often the location for crime, vandalism, sexual activity, and anti-social behavior. Government-supported schools are preventing students from using lavatories. Transit systems have put their amenities off limits to passengers.

"Part of the problem is that public toilets are not often regarded as priorities: they are often seen as amenities rather than necessities... and cost (as related to security and maintenance expenses) is another issue" (Brubaker, 2007).

By contrast, public toilets in the Far East are seen as an essential and integral component of good urban design and a cultured, civilized society. They are respected landmarks and sources of civic pride. Pioneering efforts are already underway to improve public restrooms in some of Asia's largest cities. For example, the People's Republic of China spent millions upgrading public lavatories in preparation for the Beijing 2008 Summer Olympics: it is said the city has the most public toilets of any city in the world with more than 5,000 public toilets built and renovated ("Beijing", 2008). Japan is considered the home of the futuristic commode: its toilets boast many advanced high-tech features, some of which sell for thousands of dollars. With a goal of water conservation, many of the new low-flow models use just 20% the water that conventional toilets do (Hall & Tashiro, 2007).

For us paruretics, the need to educate professionals in bathroom design is critical. Architects, facilities managers, and building code officials must be encouraged to provide environments that are sensitive to our privacy and territory needs through the use of visual barriers, sound barriers, and aesthetic layouts, and with cleanliness, hygiene, and sanitation issues as priorities. Developing worldwide standards that incorporate these needs and components would facilitate consistent bathroom design, increasing the number of public facilities that would successfully be used by the millions of paruretics who are not able to use many of those in existence today.

To advocate for improved restroom design, contact the American Restroom Association, an IPA subsidiary, at:

American Restroom Association
P.O. Box 65111
Baltimore, MD 21209
202-470-3011
www.americanrestroom.org

Gender Equity in Bathrooms (aka "Potty Parity")

"Women need more restroom facilities simply because women take longer" (CNN, 2003) is the essence of what has come to be known as restroom equity, or in its less sanitized version as *potty parity*. Potty parity legislation, which is increasingly being adopted around the country, is designed to end the long lines which form outside female restrooms in many public places by mandating additional outlets for females.

Research studies have confirmed that women take about twice as much time as men to use restroom facilities. In a groundbreaking 1988 dissertation thesis, Sandra Rawls, of Virginia Polytechnic Institute, actually timed men and women outside restrooms. She discovered that whereas men took only about 84 seconds, women took almost three minutes (Swisher, 1989). She concluded that it takes longer for women to use the restroom "not because they spend too much time fussing in the mirror, but because there are fewer facilities for them to use, even when the square footage of women's and men's rooms are equal" (Ford 2005).

John Banzhaf III, a public interest law professor at George Washington University Law School, has been a major force behind state legislation to increase the ratio of women's toilets to men's in public restrooms in order to shorten lines for women. He writes:

> The issue of restroom equity arises in part from the custom – often dictated by building-design considerations – of making men's and women's restrooms of equal size. Since at least two urinals usually can fit in the floor space required for each toilet stall, men's restrooms frequently have a larger number of facilities (urinals and toilets) than do women's. Thus, even the provision of an equal number of facilities, rather than simply equal floor space, would still result in considerably longer waits in women's restrooms if demand is comparable (Banzhaf, 1990).

Adds Mary Anne Case, a University of Chicago School of Law professor who researches regulations of sex and gender, "more space in the women's washroom is given to mirrors, grooming areas and amenities like couches, relegating the necessary fixtures to an even smaller space." (Whitacre, 2004).

The absence of potty parity can be observed readily at places of assembly, such as theaters and entertainment arenas, stadiums, airports, bus terminals, convention halls, amusement facilities, fairgrounds, zoos, colleges, and specialty events at public parks. "Whenever crowds of people need to use the restroom *at the same time* – such as when an airplane arrives or during intermission at a concert – women are forced to wait in long lines to use restrooms while their male counterparts enter and leave in a flash," notes Kathryn Anthony (Mitchell, 2004).

Current laws require a 1:1 ratio of male and female restrooms in public buildings. Proponents of potty parity legislation (sometimes referred to as the Bathroom Bill of Rights or Women's Restroom Equity Bill) want to see the ratio adjusted to at least two women's restroom facilities for every one of the men's.

They are succeeding, at least to some extent. "As of 2006, more than 20 states and a number of municipalities have passed laws requiring the doubling, tripling and even quadrupling of the ratio of women's-to-men's toilets in public buildings" (Mitchell, 2004).

However, while substantial progress is being made, it should be noted that the nature of potty parity laws differs in various states, and "almost all apply only to new construction or major renovations of large public buildings in which at least half the building is being remodeled. Still, while the *quantity* of available toilet stalls has improved, the *quality* of restrooms has not necessarily followed suit" (Anthony, 2007, p. 278).

[The issue of potty parity was revisited in early 2007 when Nancy Pelosi was elected the first female speaker of the House of Representatives. Male representatives have a fancy multi-stall bathroom with a shoeshine man, fireplace, and a television right outside the chamber's door. The closest women's restroom is far from the House floor and requires all 71 female members to either maneuver through tourist crowds or take a shortcut through the minority leader's office, navigate a corridor that winds past secretarial desks, and punch a keypad code to gain restricted access to three stalls (Talev, 2006)].

Female paruretics would likely benefit by having more stalls available, thus reducing or eliminating waits in line to use them. If men and women are to have equal wait times, it would seem women's restrooms must be far larger than men's rooms and have substantially more toilets than the total number of toilets and urinals in the men's room.

Further legislation needs to be enacted that would provide equal speed of access to public restrooms for men and women and make it mandatory that large buildings and public spaces have at least a 2:1 ratio of women's to men's restrooms.

Increasing Popularity of Unisex or Gender-Neutral Restrooms in America

In recent years, the popularity of gender-specific single-person restrooms with lockable doors has grown in the U.S. This type of facility typically has a toilet and wash basin (but also may contain a urinal) and is distinctly marked "women" and "men."

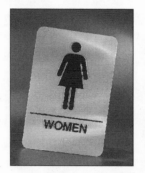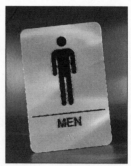

These signs can be found in airports, medical centers, parks, and small businesses.

Sex-separated public washrooms, however, have been found to intimidate transgender or androgynous people, who are often subject to embarrassment, harassment, or even assault or arrest by others offended by the presence of a person they interpret as being of the other gender. As a result of several campaigns initiated by transgender organizations and student activists, many men's and women's facilities have given way to "de-gendered" restrooms, devoid of urinals as well as male or female pictograms of white stick figures with pants or a skirt. In fact, 54% of the country's top 25 universities now have gender-neutral bathrooms, according to a study by the Gender Public Advocacy Coalition (Gender PAC) released in August 2007 (Hollenbeck, 2007).

A gender-neutral or de-gendered washroom is a single-person facility which is not labeled male or female but rather is available to everyone, no matter what their gender or biological sex.

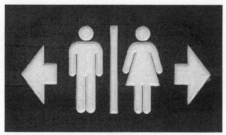

Common in several European and some Asian countries for years, they may reflect a change in attitudes and habits and are starting to replace or augment the traditional "his or hers" restrooms.

Source: www.AIGA.org

Public domain

Single person, gender-neutral washrooms have become a good solution to ensure access and to eliminate barriers for all, no matter what their gender, physical ability, health status, or level of shyness. They also address problems that parents with small children and opposite-sex caregivers face. This is not to say traditional bathrooms are being removed, but simply that additional gender-neutral bathrooms also are becoming available (for a directory, consult www.safe2pee.com). Some businesses and organizations are voluntarily converting multi-stall bathrooms into gender-neutral ones, leaving at least one men's and women's room in the building. According to the 2007 Gender Issues in the Workplace Survey by career publisher Vault Inc., a high percentage (51%) of workplaces have single-occupancy bathrooms that are open to both sexes ("Unisex Bathrooms", 2007).

The next frontier may be gender-neutral multi-person washrooms, signaling a further change in social attitudes. Co-ed bathrooms, of course, have become a fixture on many college campuses. The younger generation is far more likely to challenge the long-cherished assumptions about the benefits of sex segregation in bathrooms.

The idea of a unisex workplace bathroom, with men and women urinating side-by-side, was introduced to popular culture by the *Ally McBeal* television show in the 1990s, where it became a signature feature and seemed to represent the cutting edge of social change.

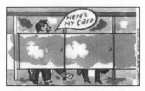

Reprinted with permission
of the illustrator,
Michael Zaharuk

In terms of public restrooms, one solution, it would seem, is to design facilities that would provide a higher level of personal privacy in each stall – separate cubicles with no gaps and strong, effective locks – combined with a common area equipped with sinks and mirrors for use before and/or after. Some European countries already provide separate ceiling-to-floor lockable rooms on one side, with a common bank of sinks on the other side.

Combining men's and women's bathrooms would result in greater efficiency in terms of use of space and maintenance. In the long term, building owners would save money in new construction costs because they could build one bathroom and install one set of sewer and water lines instead of two.

Gender-neutral multi-stall bathrooms would also help to reduce unequal bathroom lines – men and women would wait in line for the same length of time, alleviating the longer lines at women's bathrooms.

By eliminating urinals, egalitarian bathrooms might be a good idea for anyone with strong privacy needs. Some male paruretics would benefit from having private cubicles, removing the stigma that many feel is attached to using them. Females, whether paruretic or not, however, may not feel safe sharing a public restroom with males. For paruretics whose main concern is feeling pressured about time, egalitarian bathrooms might create additional stress. It appears that, for a variety of reasons, most people in the United States are not ready to accept mixed-sex provision of bathrooms, and controversy swirls around the idea.

Female Urinal Fixtures (permanent facilities)

Equally controversial is the topic of stationary floor and wall-mounted female urinals for women. These differ from the portable urinals used in lieu of bedpans, by partially immobilized people, or for purposes of travel.

As discussed in Appendix 1, urination history reveals that men and women have had different urinating positions in different cultures and have exchanged positions over time; for periods of time, female urinals were commonplace.

It is noteworthy that in certain countries, particularly western ones, modern women have, by and large, steadfastly resisted the notion of a fixed female urinal. Yet studies have shown that many, concerned about bacterial contamination from toilet seats as well as lack of hygiene, don't sit on the toilet seat anyway – up to 85% of British women, according to a 2006 study by the Chartered Society of Physiotherapy (Chartered Society, 2006) and 92% of French women, according to a poll conducted by the French Institute of Public Opinion (IFOP) (Urinelle, n.d.).

Rather than standing at a urinal or sitting on a toilet seat, many women adopt a squatting position, semi-sitting or hovering over the toilet. While this position has merit hygienically, it may result in the bladder not fully emptying. This practice can lead to urinary tract infections (UTIs) and over the long term result in compromised normal bladder function (Chartered Society, 2006).

In reality, toilet seats shouldn't be feared. One study, conducted by Dr. Charles Gerba, an environmental microbiologist from the University of Arizona and a leading expert on domestic and public hygiene, revealed that the toilet seat is actually the cleanest part of the bathroom after the sink ("ABC News", 2005).

The 1930s

Female urinals are not new to western culture. Early attempts were made in Britain in the late 1920s and early 1930s to market a urinal for women that would allow them to urinate from a standing position, without the need to sit on a shared seat.

They were introduced into the United States from Europe in the early 1930s (along with the bidet, which is still being made), and were intended as a convenience for women who did not want their bodies coming into contact with dirty public toilet seats.

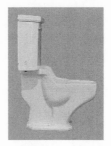

Ancient female urinal

Reprinted with permission of Adam Zieve at Square Deal and Bob Payne at Debbies Book http://www.debbiesbook.com/files/x/a0216/

The wall-mounted ones looked very much like men's urinals, and could be used either with stalls or lined up like their male counterparts. Basically the urinals featured a protruding narrow bowl that the user was expected to straddle while facing the wall, having first lowered her underpants and hiked up her skirt.

These units were male attempts to make women's public restrooms more efficient. This first wave of urinals did not catch on because of their "alien" design.

The 1950s

The next wave of female urinals was introduced in the early 1950s and installed in "heavy use" institutions, such as national park and zoo restrooms and university campuses.

Popular toilet maker manufacturer American Standard developed a product called the *Sanistand*™, and Kohler introduced its product, *Hygeia*™.

"Advertising for *Sanistand*™ made no reference to space-efficiency or cost; rather, American Standard attempted to sell the fixture to women with the promise that they didn't need 'to sit or touch [it] in any way,' playing on fears of contagion and implicitly acknowledging that then, as now, the majority of women prefer to hover when using public toilets" (Penner, Fall 2005).

There are leftovers of those fixtures still to be found installed around the United States. The one pictured here is in the Smithsonian.

A similar fixture was produced by Japanese toilet maker manufacturer TOTO from 1951 to 1971; in fact, it appeared in a bathroom for female athletes during the 1964 Summer Olympics in Tokyo.

Because these devices were not perceived to offer any real advantage over conventional toilets and also used many gallons of water per flush, they never were widely accepted. They were perceived to be awkward to use and had a lot of "splash back."

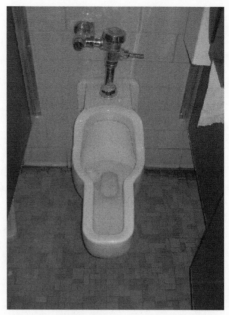

Sanistand **woman's urinal at the Smithsonian**

Image Copyright 2000-2007 www.urinal.net

The 1990s

During the early 1990s, manufacturers launched newer designs for female urinals. In 1991, a woman in Florida developed a female urinal to eliminate long lines and health risks in overcrowded ladies' rooms. Called the *She-inal*™ and manufactured by Urinette, it resembles a urinal for men, but has a hose attached and is enclosed by partitions.

The *She-inal*™ shown below is ranked number six on the list of the top 10 urinals in the world, according to one popular website (www.urinal.net).

The rationale governing its design was that because the cubicles are narrower than traditional toilets, more could fit into the same space, and because users do not have to undress as much, the process would be quicker and thus, lines would move faster.

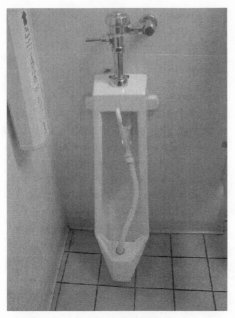

Like its predecessors, the *She-inal*™ did not prove popular. The invention was problematic because it required women to press a communal funnel-like plastic piece against their genital area.

By the late 1990s, other manufacturers sought to develop a functional, sensible, and aesthetically-pleasing female urinal that would allow more hardware into a given restroom space and cut down on the time required to enter and exit a standard toilet stall.

She-inal™
in a Dairy Queen Restaurant.
in Port Charlotte, FL

Image © 2000-2007 www.urinal.net

In March 1999, the *Lady P*™ female urinal was introduced by a Dutch bathroom equipment firm, N.V. Royal Sphinx Gustavsberg.

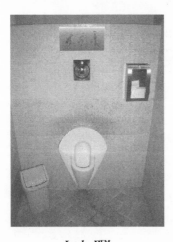

Designed for the female anatomy and considered more hygienic because a woman doesn't sit on it, the *Lady P*™ consists of a ceramic pot, a frosted partition wall, space for a toilet paper dispenser, and a disposal unit, as well as storage hooks or shelves for handbags and jackets.

Women are supposed to hover over and urinate into the *Lady P*™ bowl from on high, in a sort of a contact-free "skiing" position.

Lady P™

Image © 2000-2007
www.urinal.net

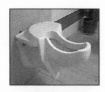

Lady Loo™
Goh Ban Huat Berhad

www.gbhgroup.com
my/saniware/saniware4c

Malaysia-based GBE introduced a similar product, the *Lady Loo™*, at about the same time that the *Lady P™* made its debut. The *Lady Loo™* fixture features a curved bowl.

The new millennium

 In March of 2006, the *Uni-Pee®*, a co-ed urinal, was introduced by Tamar Dax, a design student and winner of the prestigious Red Dot award in the international design competition of 2005.

The *UniPee®* designed by Tamar Dax – www.yankodesign.com

A cross between a conventional toilet and a urinal, the *Uni-Pee®* is meant to serve both genders; men can use it standing and women can use it in a semi-squat. It was designed to address issues of cleanliness and maintenance within technological limitations and ergonomic feasibility.

A growing number of high-end urinals are now finding a home in residential bathrooms, particularly in luxury master suites and powder rooms. Some have a distinctly feminine appeal. Marketers focus on claims about cleanliness in an effort to overcome negative associations and also stress environmental benefits (Gannon, 2007). It is too premature to predict whether their popularity will transcend the sexes so that women will adopt them for their own use, though such acceptance seems doubtful.

Not catching on

It appears that none of these contemporary female urinals, as currently designed, will receive popular support. There are three reasons:

1. Most importantly, women in western countries are naturally unaccustomed to urinating while standing up. They are not taught how to control their sphincter muscles so as to urinate without also defecating as is the common practice in some non-western countries. This can be attributed to lack of knowledge and societal conditioning that suggests there is only one "right" way for a woman to urinate. Many women refuse to use a female

urinal not on practical grounds but because to use it feels immodest or unnatural or just simply weird. Many of our toilet attitudes and habits form during in childhood and, some argue, are fundamental to our gendered sense of self.

2. The female urinals that heretofore have been developed require women to back on to the unit and adopt the traditional position of hovering/squatting rather than facing it directly. This can be very uncomfortable, stressful (especially for older or pregnant women), and potentially debilitating.

3. Women may not know what a female urinal is and how to use one. Many look like a wall-hung bidet-style toilet bowl over which the user hovers. Not surprisingly, they have sometimes been mistaken as conventional toilet bowls with imaginably disastrous results.

In order for female urinals to be totally accepted, the critical issue of woman standing and urinating has to be addressed. Women possess the physical ability to do so. Scientific studies have demonstrated that a woman can, in fact, urinate standing up, probably as well as a man, provided that she tilts her pelvis. Writes Professor Alexander Kira, "...for all practical purposes, she has little control over the direction of the urine stream in the customary assumed sitting posture. In a standing position, however, a fair degree of control is possible by projecting the pelvis forward or backward" (Kira, p. 143).

To urinate from a standing position, women must undergo a complex sort of retraining, one that reverses or subverts the socialization process. It does seem that the concept of women standing to urinate is beginning to be adopted by some women, particularly younger ones, for multiple reasons.

o Changes have been made in the design of female underwear, including unisex underwear, and also in the design of specialist outdoor clothing that offers zippers for women so they can urinate while standing without any undergarment inconvenience.

o Inexpensive portable prosthetic devices on the market, such as the *P-Mate*™ and other funnels and cones, can help women direct their urine stream. Such devices are being used in increasing number to facilitate upright urination.

o Websites and blogs on the subject of women standing to urinate are appearing in greater number. Survey results from one – a study conducted by Denise Decker, a registered nurse, director of a nursing home health agency and a strong proponent of the standing-up-to-urinate approach – revealed that the majority of 600 respondents indicated a desire for a female urinal where a woman would stand (Levinson, 1999).

Advantages to consider

Several advantages to the use of female urinals need to be considered. As a matter of economic reality, they are cheaper to build, cheaper to use (water usage), make more efficient use of space, are quicker for users (increased throughput), and require no touching. The installation of female urinals would:

- o Save in manufacturing costs over regular female toilets, which are used far more often for urination than defecation, and are less expensive to install in terms of pipe work.

- o Reduce water consumption globally in a society that is beginning to embrace the need to "save the planet." Multiple surveys show that a women may flush a toilet twice, before and after usage, sometimes even four times. An estimated 20% of the world's available drinking water is flushed down the toilet.

- o Decrease the amount of time spent in a regular stall, as well as cutting down the lines that form to use them (Levinson, 1999).

New ergonomically-sound, compact, and visually-appealing female urinals could be created to meet the needs of women who are willing to use them. The redesign of women's restrooms to accommodate these fixtures would take up less space and, combined with better training in how to urinate in a standing position, might result in improved public restroom facilities for all women.

Assuming the urinals would be placed in separate, individual, lockable cubicles, the impact on female paruretics who require privacy would be negligible. However, as a secondary effect, the space-saving aspect might result in shorter lines at the restroom.

Mobile Urinals for Women: Wave of the Future?

Very recently, a new version of female urinals has appeared at European and Australian musical festivals. The technology tackles the age-old problem of long waiting lines in female bathrooms. It is designed to be used in conjunction with devices such as the previously described *P-Mate*™, the disposable cone-shaped receptacle that allows women to urinate while standing. So, unlike the fixtures of old, this one requires women to assume a "standing and *facing* position" to use it.

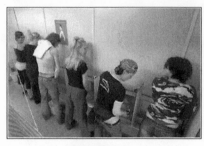

The WC1®

In the 1990s, Moon Zijp, the Dutch woman who developed the *P-Mate*™, helped create the *WC1®* (WC stands for water closet) urinal. It allows 16 women to urinate at the same time while standing upright.

In 2001, Moon Zijp pioneered the *WC2®*, which made its debut at Pinkpop, a major music festival in Amsterdam. It introduced the world to the concept of "duo-peeing." Allowing "mixed" couples to urinate together, it immediately triggered passionate discussions about women voiding like men.

Next, Moon Zijp joined forces with a manufacturer of well-known mobile urinals for men, called the *Kros Mobile Urinal®* (http://www.patent7000.com).

Together they produced the *WC3*, a plastic semi-permanent urinal that is especially adjusted to women. These urinals are grouped in fours with dividing partitions between each one. In June of 2004, this facility, dubbed the *Shee-pee®*, premiered at the Glastonbury Festival to great acclaim in the United Kingdom. This latest version featured the use of special pink-colored, female-only toilets.

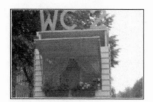

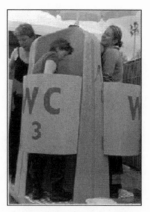

**The WC2® (above) and WC3®
(right)**

Reprinted with permission of
J.O.E Product Promotions

The concept seems to be catching on and is spreading across continents. On January 30, 2005, *Shee Pees*® were introduced in Australia at the Big Day Out musical festival in Melbourne. The following year, in February of 2006, they were used at a boutique musical festival in Stradbally, Ireland.

The key to the success of these facilities may be that women are provided with complimentary *P-mates*™ but may also be attributed to changing attitudes, especially among young women, toward using urinals.

While they may represent the wave of the future for many women, they are probably a female paruretic's worst nightmare.

Automatic Flush Toilets – They Too Can Misfire

Touch-free fixtures (including automated toilets, faucets, and soap and towel dispensers) are being introduced in new and renovated women's restrooms throughout the United States, ostensibly to conserve water and make restrooms cleaner. Patrons seem to like them because they are sanitary; janitors like them because they are easy to clean, and managers appreciate the cost savings they can provide.

Automatic flush toilets operate by sensors. The infrared devices respond to stimuli, such as motion or light, to operate the touch-free system. Standing in front of the toilet, a person reflects some of the infrared laser beam, and the autoflush device receives the reflected light. When the person moves out of the beam's path for more than three seconds, and the sensor no longer receives reflected light, the toilet flushes.

So if someone bends down to get something from a backpack or purse or just moves around too much on the toilet, s/he moves out of the infrared beam's path. The toilet thinks you left, and it goes ahead and flushes while you're still sitting on it. The result? Suddenly, one hears a sucking sound, swirling water splashes, almost "out of control," and a whooshing occurs from underneath. Sometimes these high-tech toilets become overexcited and flush themselves several times even before you even sit down, multiple times during one use, or at inopportune moments.

The toilet also may not flush when you sit on it for too long, almost as if it has lapsed into a coma, and you find yourself waving your arms in an effort to revive it. If that happens, you can press a black or rubber manual override button, if it is available, that is flush with the mechanism in order to activate it.

While automatic flushing toilets may be wonderful for keeping restrooms clean, they can also be very intimidating to paruretics (and children, as well) who may already be highly sensitized to noise and startle easily while seated on a toilet. Short of learning to dodge the laser beams, you can now purchase a device that controls automatic flush toilets. For further information about the *Flush Stopper*™, go to www.flush-stopper.com/what.html.

Eliminating Noise in a Women's Public Restroom

The Japanese experience with The Sound Princess™

Many Japanese women are embarrassed at the thought that someone else can hear them while they are doing their business on the toilet.

To cover the sound of bodily functions, many women in Japan flush public toilets continuously while using them, wasting a large amount of water in the process.

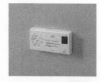

As education campaigns did not stop this practice, a device was introduced in the 1980s that, after activation, produces the sound of flushing water without the need for actual flushing.

An *Otohime*™
in a women's room

Reprinted with
permission of Toto Ltd.

One brand name commonly found is the *Otohime*™, which literally means *Sound Princess*.

This device is now routinely placed in most new public women's rooms, and many older public women's rooms have been upgraded. The *Otohime*™ may be either a separate battery-operated device attached to the wall of the toilet, or included in an existing *Washlet*™, a Japanese product that features an innovative toilet seat with an integrated bidet.

The woman activates the device by pressing a button, or by waving her hand in front of a motion sensor. After activation, the device creates a loud flushing sound similar to a toilet being flushed. This sound either stops after a preset amount of time or can be halted with a second press on the button. It is estimated that this saves up to 20 liters of water per use. However, some women believe that the *Otohime*™ sounds artificial and prefer to use a continuous flushing of the toilet instead of the recorded flush of the *Otohime*™.

Interestingly, there appears to be no demand for these devices for men's public toilets, and the devices are rarely installed in men's restrooms ("Toilets in Japan", n.d).

For female paruretics who are bothered by the sounds that others or that they themselves may (or may not) make in the toilet, the introduction of sound reduction devices such as those used in Japan would probably be a godsend.

Appendix 3
More about Author's Experience with Paruresis

By society's standards, I am probably considered a success. I have been professionally employed, worked and lived in the San Francisco Bay Area exclusively, and I own my own home. I am blessed with good friends, relatively good health, and a successful long-term relationship. I have a wide variety of interests, ranging from tennis, to the performing arts, to computers, travel, and social activism.

Despite my limitations in not being able to urinate "like everyone else," I resisted the temptation to surrender to paruresis. Instead I continued to live my life as best as I could.

I'm on the quiet, reserved, sensitive side, prone to introspection and reflection. I particularly enjoy one-on-one conversations and value simplicity and unpretentiousness. Friends might characterize me as being "nice," loyal, and responsible. Perhaps that is due to my lifelong pattern of being a people-pleaser, accommodating to the needs and wants of others in order to win their acceptance and approval, or caring too much about what others think of me.

Like many "highly sensitive people," I'm a bit of a worrier and can easily find myself feeling overwhelmed or vaguely anxious, particularly about whether I can get everything done. I prefer to "recharge my batteries" alone or in silence and like to take my time making decisions.

I consider myself a perfectionist, holding high standards for myself and others, which often gets me into trouble. At the same time, however, I have a feisty, stubborn, tenacious but lighthearted side, qualities that have allowed me to succeed and ultimately enabled me to overcome my battle with paruresis.

Origin of my problem: the teen years

My first experience with shy bladder began when I was 13 years old. Away at a family summer camp at which I had stayed for the previous 10 years, I was suddenly and inexplicably unable to urinate in a communal bathroom. Eventually I was able to, but not until well into the evening.

The next summer, at this very same camp, I again could not urinate. Only this time the consequences were more serious. My parents drove me to a hospital some distance away where I was catheterized for the first time. It hurt. Because I was menstruating at the time, I remember being tremendously embarrassed. I had to forfeit some enjoyable activities with other teens for a day until I could relax enough to void. Moreover, I carried the problem home with me, much like a leech that had attached itself and would not release its grip.

From then on, my condition took on a life of its own. Within the next few months, a number of similar incidents occurred in which I was unable to urinate: a trip to Disneyland by train, a slumber party, an overnight at my uncle's, a wisdom tooth extraction that required hospitalization. There were times when I had to ask my parents and grandmother, with whom I shared one bathroom, to leave the premises so I could "try" to relax enough to urinate. When I couldn't, I was taken to a doctor or emergency room for catheterization.

My parents, desperate for some help, took me to physicians for tests. One doctor stuck a cold, metal rod up my vagina, which really hurt. Another suggested kidney tests, during which I was injected with dye and experienced a lot of pain. A third recommended that I run water, take a warm bath or defecate in order to produce a state of relaxation. A urologist comforted my mother: *"She'll be okay once she gets married."* (It is interesting that so many doctors/mental health professionals think that paruresis may be tied to a fear of sexuality.)

Every test confirmed that the problem was mental, not physical. I was given a prescription for Librium™, a mild tranquilizer, to quell my anxiety. Sometimes this medication was effective in helping me relax enough to urinate, but many times it was not.

Arriving at college my freshman year, I spent the first week in the student health center, unable to urinate. Separated from my parents for the first time and in new surroundings, I found it difficult to cope. It took some time before I finally grew accustomed to sharing a restroom with the rest of my dorm-mates.

What was going on in my body and mind?

When I was heavily stressed and/or afraid, the tension I felt was channeled to and registered in my pelvic region. It became the repository for the expression of powerful emotions: anger, fear, and excitement. The sphincter muscles, which govern the release of urine, shut down, rendering it impossible for me to urinate except through catheterization or in the privacy of my home without anyone present. Situations that typically provoked stress for me have included being in a new environment, starting a new relationship with a male partner, traveling, being away from home, undergoing surgery, having to produce urine specimens, and feeling pressured for time.

The interior of my mind contained a constellation of restrictive thoughts which fed upon each other. I worried about someone seeing me go to the bathroom, invading my personal space, or approaching the stall in which I sat. I was overly concerned about what others were thinking about me, the negative judgments they might make. I was afraid they would become annoyed or inpatient if I took too long. They might harass or yell at me, further pressuring me to hurry up. Prior to using a restroom, my nervous system was aroused and heart rate became elevated. When I could not perform, I beat myself up. The anticipation of failure before I entered a restroom set the tone for my experience.

Young adulthood and beyond: Telling others and traveling

After graduating from college, I launched a career as a marketing analyst. Interestingly, over the years I had fewer problems urinating in work environments than in others. I cannot easily account for this phenomenon, except to speculate that I felt comfortable with the regular routines I established and was not under time pressure. Before I started a new job, I consciously checked out the location and condition of the restroom facility. Generally, I tried to time my visits so that I would be alone there.

With female friends and family members, I made it a point early on to disclose my condition, just as I had done in high school and college. While deeply embarrassed and ashamed about my condition, I adopted a matter-of-fact, positive attitude in presenting it: some people develop migraine headaches when tense, others abdominal distress, my affliction was paruresis. I really never felt judged when I revealed my "*secret*" to them; on the contrary, I felt their compassion. In telling, I removed a lot of pressure from myself. People could understand my reasons for not accompanying them to restrooms, why I found it difficult to travel, and why I sought out private restrooms.

Also, by revealing my vulnerability, others seemed to want to share something equally personal about themselves – and that built trust.

With men, I was a lot more hesitant and lacking in confidence. In simple dating relationships, I didn't feel a need to reveal my condition. Once a relationship deepened, and I began spending more time with my partner, I felt compelled to tell, mostly out of necessity. I found it difficult to participate in activities that took me away from home for a day, such as river rafting, hiking, or skiing. I also became very tense in my efforts to want to "please" and be "the perfect person." In those states, my bladder muscles involuntarily tightened and, not surprisingly, I could not urinate other than through catheterization.

In my 20s, I began a love affair with travel, whether local, domestic, or international, which has continued to the present. The relationship, though, was one of love-hate, since my symptoms became most acute when I ventured away from home. Despite having paruresis, I made the conscious decision to not let it prevent me from exploring the world. I gave myself a choice: I could either stay at home and obsess, or I could refuse to be the victim of my disability and take some risks.

I took my first international trip with a boyfriend, long before the days when my thoughts about paruresis became obsessive. The flight was delayed for many hours. After 30 hours since last voiding, I was in real pain and felt totally helpless. I notified a female flight attendant of my plight, and the pilot radioed ahead for medical assistance when the plane landed for re-fueling. Upon landing, the flight attendant announced over the loudspeaker "this airplane is now *quarantined* until one of our passengers leaves." As I was escorted down the aisle, I felt the gaze of all eyes in my direction. I felt so ashamed and embarrassed that I wanted to crawl under a seat and magically disappear.

Nevertheless, I continued to travel for the next 30 years. Group travel was especially arduous as women would descend on a restroom in herd-like fashion, and sometimes "restrooms" would consist of a hole in the ground! I didn't even bother trying; rather I sneaked off to locate a private bathroom or else held in my urine for the entire day. In between, I would worry incessantly, eliminating any pleasure I might have otherwise felt.

It was very difficult for me to have a traveling companion, to share a bathroom with a friend or acquaintance. Unwilling to abandon the pursuit of travel, I often opted for solo vacations, both domestic and international. Although I still felt a high level of anxiety prior to each trip and could not use the airport restroom before boarding an airplane, I felt confident that I could urinate in the privacy of my own bathroom – and I did. Even though I was occasionally lonely and wanted companionship, I enjoyed the freedom of being able to travel at my own pace and on my own schedule.

How I coped

My coping mechanisms have varied over the years. Beginning in my teens, I deliberately limited and cautiously monitored my fluid intake. I carefully planned trips to public restrooms based on the presence or absence of other girls and women. If they appeared, I often would "wait it out" until their departure. Noises – people talking, fans blowing, music playing, kids crying – made it difficult for me to void. A stranger or even a friend in an adjacent stall or standing in front of an occupied one made it impossible. If I observed a waiting line to use a stall or a woman taking forever to apply her make-up, I would immediately walk out the door. I searched for a private sanctuary in which to relax and take as much time as I needed.

I learned to use handicapped private restrooms when they were available. I held my urine for long periods of time despite the knowledge I might be causing damage to my body. I urinated as much as possible when at home and before leaving my home. I tried using distraction techniques, such as working on a crossword puzzle or reviewing my calendar, while seated on a toilet. Sometimes that process provided enough stimulus for my bladder to empty.

I continued to rationalize away my condition and accept my fate and circumstances. "Some people, I told myself, are in wheelchairs, while others are blind. They manage, you can, too." In the most desperate of times, I prayed.

I have been catheterized innumerable times in my life, by physicians, nurses, even boyfriends. Later, I learned to catheterize myself, which, while providing immediate relief, did not necessarily end my mental turmoil.

As the years wore on, I became increasingly paralyzed, barely able to perform this natural physical act. My coping strategies began to fail. My bladder capacity, for example, diminished over time, and I could no longer hold my urine for excessive periods of time without feeling pain.

The Valium™ that I had been ingesting in increasing dosages to help me relax so that I could urinate made me sleepy and affected my ability to concentrate.

More importantly, I developed a steady stream of obsessive thoughts and negative self-talk about the consequences of *not* being able to urinate, the what-ifs. What if I can't empty my bladder on this trip? How will I find help? Will I be like this for the whole trip? I will ruin it for my partner and for me, and I will be rejected. I viewed the world catastrophically, feeling little more than doom and gloom.

My fears built and built, and I could not control my ruminations. Even after a successful catheterization I could not relax my bladder muscles enough to urinate on my own, sometimes for periods of up to three days. This was a brand new development and caused me great anguish.

I started to limit my activities – something I vowed never to do – and began to further construct my life around the whereabouts of bathrooms. Trapped in a prison of my own creation, I had reached the point of no return. I wanted to end my suffering because the quality of my life had deteriorated so much.

In therapy

I tried many different kinds of therapies to help me address my paruresis over the years, but to no avail.

An advocate of personal counseling, I sought professional help whenever I endured crisis situations. These included coping with heavy loss (facing the premature death of my parents at an early age, followed by the death of my maternal grandmother), dealing with adoption issues and the search for my birthparents, coping with unexpected job losses, and handling relationship conflicts. I also participated in support groups, allowing me to share my thoughts and feelings with others in a similar position. Later, I continued traditional talk therapy, augmented by group experiences, in order to gain further insight into my behavior patterns and inner world.

While I always discussed my experience with paruresis during an intake interview, it was never the "presenting problem"; rather I mentioned it almost casually and put it on the backburner – despite the mental torture I continually endured.

I spent several sessions with various therapists reviewing my history with paruresis and examining its genesis. I approached the subject intellectually, trying to understand its meaning in my life and the purpose it served. Full of the best of intentions, therapists listened, offered suggestions, and helped me plan coping strategies (most of which encouraged avoidance).

Over the course of several years, I tried biofeedback, hypnotherapy, gestalt therapy, acupuncture, visualization, acupressure, meditation, and bioenergetics. None of these therapeutic approaches or practices helped to resolve my problem.

Learning to catheterize myself

When I wanted to learn to catheterize myself, I sought help from my family physician of many years. Worried about the risk of infection or potential damage to my urethra, he refused to teach me. After making a series of telephone calls to find out who could, I ended up at a women's feminist health collective. There a kind nurse practitioner instructed me – no questions asked.

The way in which I was taught, lying on my back while using a mirror to locate the opening of my urethra, proved detrimental in the long run. In this position I could not comfortably catheterize myself in many circumstances, such as when traveling on an airplane.

Years passed before I learned about alternative and more practical positions, such as sitting on a toilet, using a shorter catheter, and allowing the urine to drain into a toilet bowl.

The turning points

In August of 1997, I was directed by a physician friend to a website for those who suffered from "shy or bashful bladder syndrome." When I first accessed it, I was shocked and astounded to find that – for the first time in my life – I was in the company of many others. Tears streamed down my face. Reading the posts to the Discussion Board, I felt a large measure of comfort and found a whole supportive community of compatriots, all searching for resolution, willing to share their plight and resources with one another. I felt that I had come home!

Through the Board's founder, Richard Ziprin, I was put in touch with another female who had suffered as I had. In a telephone conversation she patiently answered my questions and commiserated with my plight. At last I had found a kindred spirit!

As I continued to participate in the Discussion Board, either posting or reading others' posts, my education grew and grew. This exchange resulted in the development of an on-line relationship with many of the posters, who became a sort of surrogate support group.

About this time the organization known as the International Paruresis Association (IPA) was born, and it eventually took over the operation of the Discussion Board. I bought and studied all of the literature on the subject that the IPA recommended.

I also began to read about weekend workshops that the IPA initiated strictly for paruretics, based on a technique called desensitization or graduated exposure, in which they relearned how to urinate in the presence of others. Workshop participants reported positive results. I was intrigued, yet terrified, to attend. I did not feel prepared to take that next giant leap.

Reaching the depths and finding help and hope: Using SSRIs

In 1999, I endured some difficult times in my personal and professional life and found myself spiraling downwards within a relatively short period of time. I was under an inordinate amount of stress as several events coalesced – the discovery and removal of a pre-cancerous lump in my breast, personnel changes at work, a new project I was asked to manage – and I was also profoundly affected by the tragedies at Columbine High School.

I could not easily sleep, waking up in the middle of the night with occasional panic attacks and alternating between taking over-the-counter and prescription drugs to aid me. In a state of anxiety and/or sleep deprivation, my thoughts about not being able to urinate were uncontrollable. I had vivid dreams about not being able to locate a "safe" bathroom. I began, more and more, to plan my life around my problem. I couldn't imagine being away from home for more than a few hours. When I entered the hospital for the surgical lumpectomy, my body was trembling. I felt such tension in my pelvic area that I pleaded to be catheterized.

I ended up having to cancel a much-planned three-week trip to Europe with my then fiancée and now husband.

One evening I attended a college basketball game with him and one of his male friends. It was a very exciting and close game. I could feel the tension escalate in my pelvic region as the game score was tied. Even though I hadn't drunk much liquid beforehand, I felt as if my bladder was going to explode. I made a run for the women's restroom and removed my emergency catheter kit from my fanny pack. With no private restroom available, I was forced to use a handicapped stall. I waited until the restroom was empty. Hands trembling, I tried to quickly insert the catheter and jabbed myself until blood started to appear. The problem was that because I wasn't carrying a plastic tray and could not empty directly into the toilet, I was forced to allow the urine to spill onto the floor. I was completely humiliated and exhausted, both physically and mentally.

One day after a severe middle-of-the-night panic attack, my body shaking, my eyes filling with tears, I didn't think I could go on. My coping mechanisms had collapsed. Terrified and no longer in denial about the depths to which I had plunged, I knew I had reached the nadir of my existence.

In consultation with a friend, a child psychiatrist, I took immediate action. I contacted my HMO, and, after a period of six weeks, was finally directed to a psychiatrist.

During my initial meeting with her, I was asked to describe my history. I mentioned paruresis and its effect on my life. She diagnosed my condition as clinical depression and anxiety. In order to stabilize me, she suggested a treatment program which consisted of taking Prozac™, a Selective Serotonin Reuptake Inhibitor (SSRI), in the morning complemented by a dose of Trazodone before bedtime. Trazodone hydrochloride (Desyrel™), part of another class of antidepressant medications called serotonin modulators, helps with insomnia. The psychiatrist offered me something very important – *hope*.

Though heavily resistant to taking any anti-depressant because of the stigma attached, I felt that I had no other choice.

About five or six weeks later, the black clouds started to dissipate as the medication took effect. I felt calmer, could sleep better, and grew more confident. That these drugs not only worked to decrease my state of anxiety/depression but also served to inhibit my obsessive thoughts about urinating came as a complete surprise.

In more of a relaxed state, I was able to cultivate a ho-hum attitude: it is fine if I urinate, fine if I don't. I will not be concerned about the *outcome*. With this new mindset, I began to care less and less about what others thought of me or how long it took to use a restroom. "Let them wait, I don't care. This is *my territory*," I told myself.

A few months later, I boarded an airplane, catheter kit in tow, for a week-long trip to Washington D.C. Unlike previous trips, I wasn't particularly focused on whether I could or could not void. Two hours into the flight, my fiancée nonchalantly remarked that the bathrooms on this flight, a Boeing 767, were especially nice and unusually spacious. A physician himself, he had witnessed how much paruresis had dominated my life and participated in many catheterizations along the way.

Okay, I decided. I would check out the bathrooms, something I had stopped doing years ago or used only for purposes of self-catheterization. I had a low level of urgency, having refrained from drinking liquids before the start of the trip. I made sure no one was waiting in line. I sat on the toilet for a few minutes, using my familiar distraction techniques, and all of a sudden a stream of urine flowed. Elated yet stunned, I had achieved a major breakthrough! I couldn't wait to return to my seat, giving my fiancée a thumbs up victory sign!

Attending an IPA workshop

By the time I attended my first IPA weekend workshop, I was making good progress. Nevertheless, I approached it cautiously, making sure my catheter kit was heavily stocked in case I needed to use it. I also reserved a private room in the hotel in which the workshop was held in case there was no other comfortable place for me to urinate.

The chance to share my history with other men and women who could easily relate was worth the cost of the workshop. I was profoundly affected as each participant recounted his or her saga, hearing firsthand about the terrible impact this condition had had on their lives. I noted many commonalities among both sexes, the differences largely logistical.

When it came time to tell my story, I was very tense, feeling a high level of performance anxiety. Nevertheless, the disclosures that I and others made produced a solid level of trust and comfort between us.

Workshop participants were encouraged to create a behavioral hierarchy, listing our least-feared to our most-feared restroom situations. Most of the following sessions were devoted to practicing graduated exposure exercises, in which each person would be paired with a partner of the same gender to work through his or her hierarchy, step by step.

I worked with two other female workshop participants who became my "pee buddies" for the rest of the workshop. In doing so, I provided guidance as to my boundaries: at what distance to stand or sit, the activity I wanted them to engage in while they were waiting for me, and whether or not to engage in conversation with each other. I was in control of my experience and tempo. Gradually, throughout the course of the weekend, I brought them closer and closer. By the end of my last session, I felt comfortable urinating with one of them standing at the door of my hotel bathroom.

The post-workshop experience

Back at home, I began to practice the graduated exposure exercises, building on the very foundation I had created for myself. I took baby steps, challenging myself to *face*, rather than avoid, situations that had previously been impossible. I practiced whenever and wherever I could, alone initially but never with friends.

To overcome my fear of entering a restroom with non-paruretic female friends, I made them surrogate "pee buddies" in my mind, without their knowledge. Initially I walked into a large public restroom with a friend, making sure I sat on a toilet at least five stalls apart. I instructed her not to wait for me and gave myself permission to take as long as I needed, even if that meant sitting for quite a while. More often than not, I was able to urinate, and I congratulated myself after each "victory". Even when I was unable to urinate, I congratulated myself for taking the time to practice. Over time, I moved incrementally closer and closer to my friends.

In later sessions, I brought a friend into the restroom and began to engage in casual conversation for the first time in many, many years. Another time, a different friend and I stood in a long line at a movie theater to use one of two available stalls.

I actually found myself looking forward to these practice sessions!

On long distance airplane flights, I raised the ante by choosing to stand in a line to use the lavatory rather than doing it at times when fellow passengers were likely to be watching a movie. I also successfully met the challenge of urinating on trains and small boats.

I developed a ritual of urinating in the shower each morning before I bathe. This served to relax my bladder muscles and promote self-confidence. Soon I was doing it mindlessly.

By the time I enrolled in my second IPA workshop just one year later, I had made tremendous strides. Three other women also participated, a record number. In one practice session we simulated a situation in which one woman banged on the door to my cubicle, demanding immediate entrance. My confidence had grown to the point I could easily urinate in a public restroom with others talking to one another right in front of me.

I started to feel, for lack of a better word, *normal.* I wasn't consciously thinking of urinating. I assumed I would go, and I did.

Epilogue

The last few years have been exhilarating. I consider myself to be *almost* fully recovered from paruresis to the extent that it no longer seriously affects my life. One is never fully "cured" of paruresis, rather in a state of recovery from it.

I still, however, carry my catheter kit with me, just in case. It is my security blanket.

I have yet to conquer the great outdoors. While on a safari in Africa three years ago, I found myself feeling momentarily envious of other women who urinated effortlessly behind a bush. Only this time I was able to see the humor in the situation! I marveled at how far I had traveled – 11,000 miles just to reach this destination – yet recognized it was really the journey of a lifetime. No, I couldn't empty my bladder, but this time I laughed.

Appendix 4
Useful Information about Paruresis to Bring
with You to a Health Care Professional

The level of ignorance about paruresis in the medical field is astounding, and you would be wise to read, print out, and hand to a health care professional some of the materials that are available on the IPA's website.

One of the best descriptions of the condition comes from the American Urological Association. It gives legitimacy to an affliction that some health care workers need, require, or demand before they will take you seriously.

The following article is reprinted with special permission from the American Urological Association and appears in its entirety.

from UrologyHealth.org – http://www.urologyhealth.org/
(Reviewed July, 2005)

What is Paruresis?

Paruresis, often referred to as bashful or "shy bladder" syndrome, is a phobia that involves fear and avoidance of using public bathrooms and an intermittent idiopathic form of urinary retention. The key is that it is a form of non-obstructive urinary retention. People who suffer from paruresis have trouble initiating urine in the presence of others. More accurately, paruresis is the fear of not being able to urinate without some or complete privacy, depending on the severity of the symptoms. This disorder can interfere in a person's quality of life in a number of areas. Paruretics face difficulties ranging from work problems (when they have to submit a urine analysis for drug testing) to traveling on long plane rides to every day social situations.

What Causes Paruresis?

There are many questions still to be answered about the cause of paruresis. Paruresis can afflict a toddler in preschool, a child in early or late adolescence, or even a person in mid to late adulthood. While some paruretics cannot point to any specific triggering incident, others believe their ailment was triggered by a traumatic incident that happened prior to or during adolescence including embarrassment by a parent, teasing by classmates or siblings, harassment in public bathrooms or sexual abuse.

Although many children experience such incidents (e.g., being teased by peers while trying to use a public toilet or urinal), not everyone develops paruresis. Note that it is pathophysiological in nature, and recent research in the field of neurology shows that there may be somatic as well as psychiatric components to the problem.

How Common is Paruresis?

While there is no way for certain to know how many people suffer from paruresis, surveys done over the last several decades indicate that the numbers could range from less than 1% to more than 25% of Americans. The 1994 National Co-Morbidity Survey indicated that 6.6% (17 million people) of the population has fear of using the toilet away from home[1], although it is uncertain how many of these fears were related to the difficulties initiating urinating in public bathrooms. The observed variation in these rates of paruresis is most likely related to whether significant life interference was required in order to be considered as meeting criteria for paruresis. There is no clear estimate about this disorder on a worldwide basis, though it seems to be a serious problem in many other countries.

What Symptoms Are Associated with Paruresis?

Here is one description of how paruresis operates in a person's life: After an initial unpleasant experience, the individual anticipates difficulty urinating whenever entering a bathroom. Forcible attempts to control the process fail, and associated anxiety with performance reduces the individual's chances of urinating while in a public facility. The paruretic must then adjust to the disorder by urinating as much as possible when at home, restricting the intake of fluids, locating vacant public bathrooms and refusing extended social invitations to avoid urinating away from home.

Paruretics engage in avoidance behavior, which temporarily reduces the fear associated with an inability to urinate but reinforces the phobic pattern. While some paruretics deny feeling any overt anxiety in public bathrooms and insist that they merely can't initiate urination, others do report physiological symptoms of anxiety, including heart palpitations, sweating, dizziness, faintness and shaking.

Since this topic is rarely talked about publicly, many paruretics feel that they are the only ones suffering from it. They feel ashamed of their

---

[1] Kessler, R.C., Stein, M.B., & Berglund, P. (1998). Social phobia subtypes in the national comorbidity survey. *American Journal of Psychiatry*, 155, 613-619.

disorder and become experts at hiding it from their closest friends, spouses and even their physicians. The sense of shame, humiliation, isolation and secondary depression resulting from this situation can be debilitating.

How is Paruresis Treated?

Many people with paruresis first visit a urologist to find out if there is something physically wrong with them, and it is clear that the function of a urologist is particularly important. The urologist's role is to:

1) Make certain there is no underlying physical ailment;

2) Reassure the patient that he or she is not alone;

3) Discuss behavioral approaches, such as scheduling urination, and, for men, using a private toilet rather than a urinal;

4) Teach the patient, if he or she so desires, self-catheterization; and

5) Refer the patient to a specialist in anxiety disorders for cognitive and graduated exposure therapy.

Of these five treatment methods, self-catheterization provides an immediate way to relieve patients of their problems and improve their quality of life. The minimal risk in otherwise healthy and intellectually capable individuals far outweighs the harm done by permitting continued disruption of the patient's life.

No controlled studies of the treatment of paruresis have been published. However, behavioral exposure therapy has been reported to be helpful in several case reports over the last 40 years, with either complete or partial success. Other methods that have been used in the treatment of paruresis, with mixed results, include medications, hypnotherapy, paradoxical intention, sphincter botulinum toxin injection and surgery (i.e., transurethral microwave therapy (TUMT) or transurethral resection of the prostate (TURP).

Based on a limited sample, paruretic sufferers may also benefit from adjunct drug therapy. For some, the selective serotonin reuptake inhibitors (SSRIs) have seemed to help reduce anxiety levels enough that graduated exposure therapy began to work well. However, it is important to note that the effectiveness of any drug therapy in helping people with paruresis is purely speculative at this point. Interestingly, one standard urological treatment, the prescription of alpha-blockers, has not been proven to be effective for this disorder at this time.

What Can Be Expected after Treatment?

Assuming reassurance of the common nature of this problem and the proper and effective treatment of paruresis, most people can expect significant relief of their symptoms. While the disorder may occasionally come back, the patient, when properly educated, will not be alarmed by it, and will take appropriate measures to bring it under control again. Cognitive behavioral therapy seems 80% to 90% effective for paruresis, and with adjunct drug therapy, the disease is usually kept under control.

Frequently Asked Questions

Is paruresis hereditary?

There is some evidence indicating that paruresis might be hereditary. It is important for parents to realize that if one or both have this condition, the likelihood is increased that your child or children could develop it as well.

Where can I get more information?

International Paruresis Association at www.paruresis.org

References

ABC News. (2005, October 14). Myth: Toilet Seats Are the Dirtiest Thing in the Bathroom: You Can Find More Germs on a Desktop Than a Toilet Seat. Retrieved October 11, 2006, from http://abcnews.go.com/2020/Health/story?id=1213831&page=1

Academy of Cognitive Therapy. (n.d.). Find a Certified Cognitive Therapist. Retrieved January 1, 2006, from http://www.academyofct.org/Library/CertifiedMembers/Index.asp?FolderID=1137&SessionID={51B6C27E-41E5-4562-ACB3-557E9FE14F53}&RLMsg=&SP=

American Psychiatric Association. (1994). *Diagnostic and statistical manual of mental disorders (4th ed.)*. Washington, DC.: author.

American Restroom Association. (2006). *Home page*. Retrieved January 4, 2007, from http://www.americanrestroom.org

American Restroom Association (n.d.). Who are the restroom challenged? Retrieved November 15, 2007, from http://www.americanrestroom.org/pr/who.htm

American Urological Association. (reviewed July, 2005). Paruresis. Retrieved July 2006, from http://www.urologyhealth.org/search/index.cfm?search=paruresis&searchtype=and&topic=410

Angelo, S. (2002). External incontinence devices. Retrieved September 20, 2006, from http://www.ololrmc.com/15615.cfm

Anthony, K. (2006, November). An Update on Public Restrooms in the USA. Paper presented at the 2006 World Toilet Organization Summit in Bangkok, Thailand. Retrieved July 4, 2007, from http://www.worldtoiletexpo.com/uploads/images/337/An_Update_On_Public_Restrooms_in_the_USA_-_Prof_Kathryn_Anthony1.pdf.

Anthony, K. & Dufresne, M. (2007, February). Potty Parity in Perspective: Gender and Family Issues in Planning and Designing Public Restrooms. *Journal of Planning Literature*, Vol. 21, No. 3, 267-294. Retrieved September 16, 2007, from http://jpl.sagepub.com/cgi/content/abstract/21/3/267

Anxiety Disorders Association of America. (n.d.). Getting Help: Find a Therapist. Retrieved November 19, 2007, from http://community.adaa.org/eweb/DynamicPage.aspx?Site=adaa&WebKey=ce66a0ec-3e19-437d-836b-f180fcdf6814

Aron, E. (1996). *The Highly Sensitive Person: How to Thrive When the World Overwhelms You*. New York: Carol Publishing.

Aronczyk, M. (2003, May 23). Bathroom boundaries and habits. *The Toronto Star*. Life Section, p F1

Au, C. (2007, July 31). Fighting for the right to flush. *Time Magazine*. Retrieved January 5, 2008, from http://www.time.com/time/nation/article/0,8599,1648349,00.html

Banzhaf, J.F. (n.d.). Is potty parity a legal right? Retrieved September 24, 2006, from http://banzhaf.net/docs/pparticle.html

Banzhaf, J.F. (1990, April 18). Final frontier for the law? *National Law Journal.* Retrieved May 1, 2006, from http://banzhaf.net/docs/potty_parity.html

Behind the bathroom door: new Uristat® survey shows urinary tract infections are common and painful (2002, January 24). Press release from McNeil-PPC, Inc. Retrieved March 8, 2006, from http://www.uristat.com/shorthed.htm

Beijing becomes city with world's largest number of public toilets (2008, March 4). *Beijing 2008.* Retrieved March 8, 2008, from http://en.beijing2008.cn/news/olympiccities/beijing/n214261401.shstml

Bradley, M. (2006, March). Potty parity may trim long restroom lines. *Deseret News.* Retrieved March 15, 2007, from http://findarticles.com/p/articles/mi_qn4188/is_20060312/ai_n16155061

Braverman, A. (2003, April). Unexpected expertise: Mary Anne Case – toilet inequities. *University of Chicago Magazine* April (95): 4. Retrieved April 20, 2006, from http://magazine.uchicago.edu/0304/features/index-toilet.html

Brief Relief [product illustration]. Retrieved May 18, 2006, from http://briefrelief.com/images/sub_ti_br.jpg

Brief Relief Privacy Tent. [Online Photograph]. Retrieved September 10, 2006, from http://www.westernshelter.com/prodimg.php?w=408&h=235&ID=284

Brubaker, R. & McCreary, C. (2007). Availability of restrooms in the United States and federal public health mandates: a call to action. Paper presented at the 2007 World Toilet Summit in New Delhi, India. Retrieved February 3, 2008, from www.steel-bridge.org/pdf/ARACalltoActionRBCM.pdf

CNN.com. (2003, December). NY considers women's restroom rights. Retrieved August 2006, from http://www.cnn.com/2003/US/Northeast/12/04/offbeat.rest.rooms.ap/index.html

The Chartered Society of Physiotherapy. (2006, March 8). Ladies, take a seat for International Women's Day! Retrieved October 5, 2007, from http://www.csp.org.uk/director/newsandevents/news.cfm?item_id=D537736EB3663 5EB2EA5F540CA6F9DF5

Cook, J. (2006, August). *Principles of Treatment.* Retrieved May 25, 2006, from http://www.psycserv.com/CBT_principles.htm

Crimson. (1998, August 17). Old posts from the toilet. Message posted to Toilet Stool.com. Retrieved December 5, 2007, from http://www.toiletstool.com/toilet/toiletpostcj.htm

Decker, D. (n.d.). A Women's Guide to How to Pee Standing Up. Retrieved June 15, 2007, from http://web.archive.org/web/20040213142128/http://www.restrooms.org/standing.html

Do not urinate here. [Photograph]. Retrieved September 3, 2006, from http://www.bigfoto.com/africa/ghana/ghana-66.jpg

Donovan, P. (2005, January 20). Minding their pees and queues. *The Age*. Retrieved
September 4, 2006, from http://www.theage.com.au/news/National/Minding-their-
pees-and-
queues/2005/01/19/1106110810530.html&h=165&w=200&sz=8&hl=en&start=162&si
g2=OqCeIID3X00nP7czY5_M1g&tbnid=yGAoybbJiWzcDM:&tbnh=86&tbnw=104&e
i=WFSyRqfPMIXegQOQjqGYBA&prev=/images%3Fq%3Dfemale%2Burinals%26star
t%3D160%26gbv%3D2%26ndsp%3D20%26svnum%3D10%26hl%3Den%26sa%3DN

Equality in the toilet. [cartoon]. (2003, December 4). *Eye Weekly*. Retrieved September 4,
2006, from http://www.eyeweekly.com/eye/issue/issue_12.04.03/op/editorial.php

Female urination device. (2007, June 5). In *Wikipedia, The Free Encyclopedia*. Retrieved June 1,
2006, from
http://en.wikipedia.org/w/index.php?title=Female_urination_device&oldid=136073987

The Feminal Female Urinal. [Online Photograph]. Retrieved September 10, 2006, from
http://www.brucemedical.com/femfemur.html

Female urinal from the 1930s [Online Photograph]. Retrieved September 8, 2006, from
www.debbiesbook.com/files/x/a0216/

The Flush Stopper. [Product description]. Retrieved August 6, 2007, from
http://www.flush-stopper.com/what.html

Flush toilet. (n.d.). *Wikipedia, the free encyclopedia*. Reference.com.Retrieved December 04,
2006, from http://www.reference.com/browse/wiki/Flush_toilet

Ford, A. (2005, February). Required Bathroom Reading. *Utne Reader*. Retrieved May 2007,
from www.utne.com/web_special/web_specials_2005-02/articles/11548-1.html

Foxman, B. (2002, July 8). Epidemiology of urinary tract infections: incidence, morbidity,
and economic costs. *The American Journal of Medicine*, Volume 113, Issue 1, Supplement 1,
5-13. Retrieved March 4, 2005, from
http://www.sciencedirect.com/science?_ob=ArticleURL&_udi=B6TDC-466R80S-
2&_user=10&_coverDate=07%2F08%2F2002&_rdoc=1&_fmt=&_orig=search&_sor
t=d&view=c&_acct=C000050221&_version=1&_urlVersion=0&_userid=10&md5=d
4d57c82ac2a196b1ca5d7088fcdb656

French Squat Toilet [Online Photograph]. Retrieved September 10, 2006, from
http://commons.wikimedia.org/wiki/Image:French_Squatter_Toilet.jpg#file

Freshette, the Feminine Urinary Director. [Product information]. Retrieved May 20, 2006,
from http://www.freshette.com/

Gannon, S. (2007, January 25). For the high-end bathroom, something unexpected. *The New
York Times*. Retrieved August 4, 2007, from
http://www.nytimes.com/2007/01/25/garden/25urin.html?pagewanted=print

Gibbs, R. (2004). *A Summary of Results from the Australian-based Global Internet Paruresis
(Shy Bladder) Survey*. Retrieved October 5, 2007, from
http://paruresis.org/research_results_RGibbs.htm

Greed, C. (2003). Inclusive urban design: Public toilets. Oxford: Architectural Press.

Greed, C. (2003). Public Toilets in the 24-Hour City. Paper presented at the 2003 World Toilet Summit in Taipei, Taiwan. Retrieved May 21, 2006, from http://www.worldtoilet.org/events/WTS2004/Public%20Toilets%20in%20the%2024%20Hour%20City%20-%20Dr%20Clara%20Greed.pdf

Greed, C. (2004). A Code of Practice for Public Toilets in Britain. Paper presented at the 2004 World Toilet Summit in Beijing, China. Retrieved May 20, 2005, from http://www.worldtoilet.org/articles/wts2004/A_Code_of_Practice_for_Public_Toilets_in_Britain.pdf

Hall, K. & Tashiro, H. (2007, January 2). Potty Talk from Japan [electronic version]. *Business Week, Asia edition*. Retrieved June 1, 2007, from http://www.businessweek.com/globalbiz/content/jan2007/gb20070102_511509.htm?chan=innovation_innovation+%2B+design_top+stories

Here's my card [cartoon]. Retrieved October 10, 2006, from http://www.eyeweekly.com/eye/issue/issue_12.04.03/op/photos/editorial.JPG

History of the embossed toilet. (n.d). Retrieved December 11, 2006, from http://www.victoriancrapper.com/Toilethistory.HTML

History of plumbing – Roman and English legacy. (n.d). Retrieved December 12, 2006, from http://www.theplumber.com/eng.html

History of toilets. (n.d). Retrieved September 15, 1006, from http://www.sulabhenvis.nic.in/Historyoftoilets.htm

Hollenbeck, S. (2007, December 2). His? Hers? Ours? These bathrooms serve all. *McClatchy-Tribune*. Retrieved February 1, 2008, from http://www.gpac.org/press/sj.12.02.07.html

How to urinate standing up as a female. (n.d). Wikihow. Retrieved April 5, 2006, from http://www.wikihow.com/Urinate-Standing-up-As-a-Female

Inflate-A-Potty. [Online Photograph]. Retrieved September 10, 2006, from http://us.st11.yimg.com/us.st.yimg.com/I/preparednesscenter_1959_55934203

International Paruresis Association. (1999-2008). *Home page*. Retrieved March 4, 2005, from http://paruresis.org/

Kessler, R., Stein, M.B., & Berglund, P. (1998, May). Social phobia subtypes in the national co-morbidity survey. *American Journal of Psychiatry, 155*, 613-619. Retrieved September 10, 2006, from http://ajp.psychiatryonline.org/cgi/content/full/155/5/613

Kira, A. (1976). *The bathroom, new and expanded* edition. New York: Penguin.

The Lady J Urinal. [Online Photograph]. Retrieved September 10, 2006, from http://www.little-john.com/litjon.html

The Lady Loo. [Online Photograph]. Retrieved September 14, 2006, from http://www.gbhgroup.com.my/saniware/saniware4c.htm

The Lady P female urinal. [Online Photograph]. Retrieved September 15, 2006, from http://www.urinal.net/casinotheater

Lark, S. (n.d.). *Relaxation Techniques for Relief of Anxiety & Stress* (Excerpted from *The Menopause Self Help Book*). Retrieved April 26, 2006, from http://www.healthy.net/scr/Article.asp?Id=1205&xcntr=2

Levine, D. (n.d.). *"What is the breath-holding technique? Does it work for everyone?* International Paruresis Association. Retrieved August 5, 2006, from http://www.paruresis.org/FAQ/FAQ_full.htm#witbhtdiwfe

Levinson, O. (1999). The female urinal: Facts and fables. Retrieved October 11, 2006, from http://www.femaleurinal.com/factsandfables.html

Lowe, L. (2005, November 10). No place to go. *The Coast.* Retrieved May 1, 2007, from http://www.thecoast.ca/1editorialbody.lasso?-token.folder=2005-11-10&-token.story=101011.112113&-token.subpub=

Magic Cone. [Product description]. Retrieved May 20, 2006, from http://www.magic-cone.com

Malouff, J. & Lanyon, R. (1985, April 1). Avoidant Paruresis: An Exploratory Study. *Behavior Modification*, Vol. 9, No. 2, 225-234. Retrieved March 8, 2006 from http://bmo.sagepub.com/cgi/contnet/abstract/9/2/225

The Millie Urinal. [Online Photograph]. Retrieved September 10, 2006, from http://www.valuemedicalsupplies.com/millie.htm

Mitchell, M. (2004, August 30). Authors advocate more and better women's restrooms in public facilities. *News Bureau University of Illinois at Urbana-Champaign.* Retrieved October 25, 2007, from www.news.uiuc.edu/news/04/0830restrooms.html

National Kidney and Urologic Diseases Information Clearinghouse (NKUDIC). (n.d.). *Urinary Tract Infections in Adults.* Retrieved July 30, 2005, from http://kidney.niddk.nih.gov/kudiseases/pubs/utiadult#treatment

National Kidney and Urologic Diseases Information Clearinghouse (NKUDIC). (n.d.). *Urinary Retention.* Retrieved August 4, 2007, from http://kidney.nih.gov/kudisease/pubs/UrinaryRetention/#info

National Phobics' Society (n.d.). Toilet Phobia and the National Phobics Society (NPS). Retrieved February 2, 2008, from http://phobics-society.org.uk/condition_toiletphobia.php

Nelson, K. (2003, July 29). Helping unlock the bathroom 'stall'. *Boston Globe Correspondent.* (p. c3). Retrieved April 5, 2004, from http://search.boston.com/local/Search.do?s.sm.query=Helping+unlock+the+bathroom+stall&s.author=Nelson&s.tab=globe&s.si%28simplesearchinput%29.sortBy=&docType=&date=&s.startDate=2003-07-29&s.endDate=2033-07-29

Nugent, M. (2004, September 28). No laughing matter: bashful bladder syndrome leads to social withdrawal. *New Jersey Star-Ledger.*

Odell, J. (1997). Musings of a Privy Digger. Retrieved October 10, 2006, from http://www.bottlebooks.com/privyto.htm

Paha Qué TeePee Shower and Outhouse Tent. [Online Photograph). Retrieved September 10, 2006, from http://www.pahaque.com

Paul, J. (2006). Using the Urinal Game and Other Bathroom Customs to Teach the Sociological Perspective. Electronic Journal of Sociology. Retrieved may 4, 2007 from http://72.14.253.104/search?q=cache:35sBL7HYlxYJ:www.sociology.org/content/200 6/tier2/johnpaul_the_urinal_game.pdf+Using+the+Urinal+Game+and+other+Bathro om+Customs&hl=en&ct=clnk&cd=1&gl=us&lr=lang_en&client=firefox-a

The Pee-Mate. [Product description]. Retrieved May 20, 2006, from http://www.pmateusa.com/

Penner, B. (2005, Fall). A revolutionary aim? *Cabinet* (Issue 19). Retrieved August 20, 2006, from http://www.cabinetmagazine.org/issues/19/penner.php

Penner, B. (2005, June). Researching Female Public Toilets: Gendered Spaces, Disciplinary Limits. *Journal of International Women's Studies,* 6,2, 3-5. Retrieved August 20, 2006, from http://www.iiav.nl/ezines/web/JournalofInternationalWomensStudies/2005/June/bri dgew/Penner.pdf

The PETT Toilet. [Online Photograph]. Retrieved September 10, 2006, from http://www.thepett.com/index.php?PageLayout=PRODUCTS&headerID2=36&pageI D=98

Pickering, N. (2001, November). Paruresis: the secret bathroom phobia. Paper presented at the 2001 World Toilet Summit in Singapore. Retrieved March 4, 2006, from http://www.worldtoilet.org/images/stories/WTOS2001/pickering_-_paruresis_- _the_secret_bathroom_phobia_wtos_01.pdf

Place & Process in the Ladies Room. (n.d.). *Customer Experience Crossroads.* Retrieved October 10, 2006, from http://www.customercrossroads.com/customercrossroads/2006/11/place_process_i.html

Portable toilet made of corrugated paper board. [Online Photograph]. Retrieved September 10, 2006, from http://www.outbackpack.com/img4.gif

The PUP Privacy Shelter. [Online Photograph]. Retrieved September 10, 2006, from http://www.thepett.com/images/page/page99/PUP-&-PETT.jpg

Relaxation Techniques (n.d.). Retrieved April 26, 2006, from http://www.optimalhealthconcepts.com/Stress

Research Pod (n.d.). Making a stand to take a pee. Retrieved January 1, 2006, from http://www.researchpod.com/pdf/making_a_stand_to_take_a_pee.pdf

Restop [product illustration]. Retrieved September 12, 2006, from http://restop.com/products/restop1.html

Restop Privacy tent. [Online photograph]. Retrieved September 12, 2006, from http://restop.com/products/privacy-tent.html

Roach, M. (1999, May 21). Bashful Bladders. *Salon magazine.* Retrieved November 5, 2005, from http://www.salon.com/health/col/roac/1999/05/21/shy_bladder/

Robbins, C. (2006, March 5). Running from embarrassment [Msg. 1102]. Message posted to http://www.paruresis.org/phpBB2/viewtopic.php?p=1102&highlight=#1102

Robbins, C. (2006, November 11). It's not a fear of urinating [Msg. 7494]. Message posted to http://www.paruresis.org/phpBB2/viewtopic.php?p=7494&highlight=#7494

Robbins, C. (2006, November 22). Thinking it through [Msg. 7734]. Message posted to http://www.paruresis.org/phpBB2/viewtopic.php?p=7734&highlight=#7734

Robbins, C. (2007, January 7). Positive self-talk [Msg.8540]. Message posted to http://www.paruresis.org/phpBB2/viewtopic.php?p=8540&highlight=#8540

Robbins, C. (2007, April 10).Cognitive Therapy Myths [Msg. 2389].Message posted to http://www.paruresis.org/phpBB2/viewtopic.php?t=2389

Robbins, C. (2007, May 28). Nobody notices, nobody cares [Msg.11944]. Message posted to http://www.paruresis.org/phpBB2/viewtopic.php?p=11944&highlight=#11944

Sanistand women's urinal [Online photograph]. Retrieved September 12, 2006, from http://urinal.net/national_zoo/

Schmidt, J., & Brubaker, R. (2004, November). The code and practice of toilets in the United States of America. Paper presented at the 2004 World Toilet Summit in Beijing, China. Retrieved October 11, 2006, from http://www.americanrestroom.org/wto/wts04_paper.pdf

Schuster, C. (2005). *Public Toilet Design: From Hotels, Bars, Restaurants, Civic Buildings and Businesses Worldwide.* Italy: Firefly Book, Ltd.

She-inal Dairy Queen [Online photograph]. Retrieved September 10, 2006, from http://www.urinal.net/dairy_queen/

The Shee-pee . [Online Photograph]. Retrieved September 10, 2007, from http://www.p-mate.com/eng/wc3.html

Skinner, A. (2003). *How to Pee Standing Up: Tips for Hip Chicks.* New York, NY: Simon & Schuster, Inc.

Soifer, S., Zgourides, G., Himle, J., & Pickering, N. (2001). *Shy bladder syndrome: Your step-by-step guide to overcoming paruresis.* Oakland, CA: New Harbinger.

Soifer, S. (n.d.). The Evolution of the Bathroom and the Implications for Paruresis. Retrieved April 1, 2006, from http://www.paruresis.org/evolution.htm

Stadium Gal [product illustration]. Retrieved May 18, 2006, from http://www.biorelief.com/store/stadiumgal.html#

Stansport Folding Portable Toilet. [Online Photograph]. Retrieved September 10, 2006, from http://www.epcamps.com/portable_toilet.html

Stapells, C. (1999, October 4). Pee-formance anxiety: You know you're in trouble when you can't go in a public washroom. *Toronto Sun.* Retrieved May 8, 2004, from www.canadianrockhound.com/sun/toronto_sun.html

Stoke-on-Trent City Council. (n.d.). Public Toilets: A History. Retrieved January 20, 2006, from http://www.stoke.gov.uk/ccm/museums/museum/2006/gladstone-pottery-museum/information-sheets/public-toilets.en;jsessionid=a6Oc12xCCve5

Stress Management. (n.d.). Retrieved April 26, 2007, from http://mentalhealth.about.com/od/stress/Stress_Management.htm

Swisher, K. (1989, August 10). Potty Parity. *Washington Post.* Retrieved March 1, 2006, from http://www.highbeam.com/doc/1P2-1205803.html

Talev, M. (2006, December 24). Will female speaker establish 'potty parity' in House? *Sunday Gazette-Mail*. Retrieved March 15, 2006, from http://www.highbeam.com/doc/1P2-14766960.html

Toffler, A. (1970). *Future Shock*. New York: Bantam Books.

Toilet History. (n.d). Bricks and Brass. Retrieved June 5, 2007, from http://www.bricksandbrass.co.uk/deselem/watsew/watsewtoil.htm

Toilets in Japan (n.d.). Wikipedia, the free encyclopedia. Retrieved February 2. 2006, from http://en.wikipedia.org/wiki/Toilets_in_Japan

TravelJohn [product illustration]. Retrieved May 18, 2006, from http://www.traveljohn.com/1-1-1.php

TravelJohn Privacy Shelter. [Online Photograph].Retrieved September 10, 2006, from http://www.traveljohn.com/1-1-7.php

Travelmateinfo.com. (2003). [Travelmate urinary products overview]. Retrieved June 15, 2006, from http://www.travelmateinfo.com/page002.html

Uni-Pee Co-Ed Urinal. [Online Photograph].Retrieved September 10, 2007, from http://www.red-dot.sg/concept/porfolio/winners/interior/unip.htm

Unisex Bathrooms Are No Longer a Rarity at Work. (2007, June 14). *Business Wire*. Retrieved February 15, 2008, from http://www.allbusiness.com/services/business-services/4352203-1.html

Urinelle: A new hygiene accessory for all women.(n.d). Retrieved September 10, 2007, from http://www.urinelle.biz/images/UrinelleENGLISH.pdf

Urinelle [product illustration]. Retrieved May 18, 2006, from http://www.urinelle.biz/

The WC1. [Online Photograph]. P-Company. Retrieved September 10, 2007, from http://www.p-mate.com/eng/wc3.html

The WC2 . [Online Photograph].P-Company. Retrieved September 10, 2007, from http://www.p-mate.com/eng/wc3.html

The WC3. [Online Photograph]. P-Company. Retrieved September 10, 2007, from http://www.p-mate.com/eng/wc3.html

Webber, Rebecca. (2001, July 15). Public toilets. GothamGazette.com, Retrieved June 6, 2006, from http://www.gothamgazette.com/iotw/bathrooms/

Weil, M. (2001, May). A Treatment for Paruresis or Shy Bladder Syndrome. *The Behavior Therapist*, Vol. 24, No. 5, 108.

Wells, R. & Giannetti, V. (1990). *Handbook of the Brief Psychotherapies*. New York: Plenum Publishing.

Whitacre, S. (2004, March). Restrooms: separate and unequal?. *Contracting Profits*. Retrieved February 2, 2008, from http://www.cleanlink.com/cp/article.asp?id=1163

The Whiz Freedom. [Product description]. Retrieved May 20, 2006, from http://www.whizproducts.co.uk/en/whiz_freedom.aspx

Whizzy for women. [Product description]. Retrieved May 18, 2006, from
http://www.whizzy4you.com/

Women's bathroom. [Cartoon]. Retrieved April 10, 2006, from http://www.little-john.com/litjon.html

World Toilet Organization. (2001-2008). *Home page*. Retrieved September 10, 2007, from
www.worldtoilet.org

Zahuruk, M. [cartoon]. (2003, December). *Eye Weekly*. Retrieved June 3, 1006, from
http://www.eyeweekly.com/eye/issue/issue_12.04.03/op/editorial.php

Zeff, T. (2004). *The Highly Sensitive Person's Survival Guide*. Oakland, CA: New Harbinger
Publications, Inc.

Index

A

Academy of Cognitive Therapy, 74, 165

Acceptance and Self-Appreciation, 33, 86

American Restroom Association, 132, 165

American Urological Association, 27, 161, 165

Anthony, Dr. Kathryn, 18, 128, 129, 131, 133, 165

Antibiotics. *See* Medication and drugs

Antidepressants. *See* Medication and drugs

Aron, Dr. Elaine, 28, 31, 165, *See* Highly Sensitive People

Assistive devices, 56, 57, 70, 109, 117, 120

   Disposable urinal bags, 70, 71, 117, 118

   External collection, 70, 117

   Funnels, 57, 70, 117, 120, 142

   Portable toilets. *See* Portable toilets

   Portable urinals. *See* Urinals

Automatic flush toilets, 52, 145

Avoidance of bathrooms, 1, 6, 9, 23, 27, 35, 112, 155, 161, 162

B

Banzhaf, John, 133, 166, See Potty Parity

Bathroom Bill of Rights. See Potty Parity

Bathroom design, 16, 128, 129, 132

   Flaws, 15, 113, 129

   Standards, 129, 132

Bathroom lines, 11, 17, 18, 19, 41, 132, 133, 136, 139, 143, 166

Bathrooms

   Behavior in, 16, 17, 18

   Family, 16, 129, 131

   Gender-neutral, 16, 136

   History, 125

   Sanitation and hygiene, 18, 132, 137, 140, 145

   Unisex, 58, 131, 135, 136

   User needs, 128, 132

Baumgaertner, Phil, i, vii

Behavioral therapy, 5, 73, 163

   Desensitization and gradual exposure, 73, 79, 156

   Hierarchy scales, 79, 81, 83, 85, 97, 159

   Other exposure exercises, 43, 88

   Paradoxical intention, 86

   Practice of exercises. *See* Practice

Biofeedback, 3, 94, 95, 155

Bladder dysfunction. *See* Paruresis: Physiology/bladder dysfunction

Books Recommended, 27

Breath holding, 73, 91, 108, 169

Breathing techniques, 32, 44, 88, 91

C

Case, Mary Anne, 133, 166

Catheter, 2, 7, 19, 20, 63, 64, 157, 160

Catheterization, 2, 64, 65, 150, 151, 152, *See* Clean Intermittent Self-Catheterization (CISC)

CBT. *See* Cognitive-Behavioral Therapy (CBT)

Challenge your thinking, 31, 37, 43, 47, 51, 52, 75

Clean Intermittent Self-Catheterization (CISC), 6, 19, 55, 56, 63, 64, 65, 66, 70, 80, 108, 153, 155, 163

Clothing, 17, 119, 142

Cognitive Therapy, 4, 76, 163, *See* What other people think

   Cognitive restructuring, 48, 50, 73, 74, 109

Cognitive-Behavioral Therapy (CBT), 3, 4, 28, 73, 88, 89, 108

Cook, Dr. John, 75

Coping techniques. *See* Paruresis, coping

Cystitis, 18, 69, *See* Urination tract infections (UTI)

Standing up to urinate. *See* Urination, Standing or hovering
Statistics, xv, 4, 20, 23, 31, 69, 84, 133, 135, 136, 137, 143, 162, 164
Stress reduction. *See* Relaxation and stress reduction techniques
Success and misfires, 5, 7, 84
Success stories, 103
Support groups, 89, 93, 97, 98, 101, 110
Surgery, 163

T

Telling others. See Disclosure
The Bathroom. See Kira, Dr. Alexander
Time pressures, 19, 32, 33, 41, 42, 43, 44, 56
Toffler, Alvin, 42, 172
Travel, 24, 55, 56, 58, 122, 152, 153
Treatment. *See* Paruresis, Treatment

U

Urgency levels, 82, 85, 92
Urinals for women
  Mobile, 143
  Permanent, 137, 138, 139, 141, 143
  Portable, 70, 117, 121
Urinary retention, 161, See paruresis

Urinary tract infections (UTI), 19, 68, 69, 137
Urination
  Assistive devices. *See* Assistive devices
  Outdoors, 55, 57, 71
  Standing or hovering, 57, 71, 117, 119, 127, 137, 138, 140, 141, 142, 143, 168
Urine specimen or sample, xv, 2, 112, 151
UTI. *See* Urinary tract infections

W

Weil, Dr. Monroe Weil, 91, 172
What other people think, 6, 11, 36, 47, 48, 49
Women's Forum, 29, 99, 108
Workshops, 80, 84, 97, 98, 101, 109, 110, 158, 159,
  Women's workshops, xiii, xvi, 98, 179

Y

Yoga, 32, 44, 91, 94, 95

Z

Ziprin, Dr. Richard, vii, 156

About the Author

Carol Olmert holds a B.A. from UCLA in Pre-Social Welfare. She has worked as a Market Research Analyst for large corporations and served as an Administrator for several non-profit organizations.

A recovered paruretic, she has served as a Board Member of the International Paruresis Association (IPA). Currently she is the Women's Coordinator for the IPA and also serves on its Advisory Board. She co-conducts workshops for women who want to recover from paruresis.

Carol lives with her husband in Walnut Creek, California.